Caring for Dying People of Different Faiths

Third edition

ia Neuberger

rner Chief Executive
King's Fund
London

Radcliffe Medical Press

Radcliffe Medical Press Ltd
18 Marcham Road
Abingdon
Oxon OX14 1AA
United Kingdom

www.radcliffe-oxford.com
The Radcliffe Medical Press electronic catalogue and online ordering facility.
Direct sales to anywhere in the world.

British Library Cataloguing in Publication Data

A catalogue record for this book is available from the British Library.

ISBN 1 85775 945 1

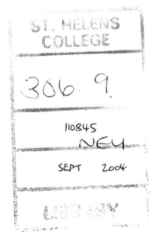
Typeset by Acorn Bookwork Ltd, Salisbury
Printed and bound by TJ International Ltd, Padstow, Cornwall

Contents

Foreword

Imagine visiting in your dreams a small world you have recently become familiar with; a world in which people of diverse faiths all receive care near the ends of their lives from one team of people. You walk into a ward of eight beds where that team is working. In one bed is someone who looks like your kid sister, now a dying young adult; you think of the work she is trying to do to help her young family survive after leukaemia takes her. In another is someone who looks familiar and he seems to be of different descent, and one of the people around him reminds you of your high school classmate. You remember conversations that helped you to understand how their faith sustained them as they missed their lost family members.

You look further and notice that everyone looks familiar yet different and you have an odd sensation that you are in the open air market not too far from your home, where people of so many ethnic, cultural and religious affiliations come to buy food and home supplies. People bustle with a sense of purpose, an edge of anxiety yet an atmosphere of life and fulfillment pervades. But here, they have come to do the work of dying. They did not come to be together. They came with a compelling need that they happen to have in common.

You start to watch the nurse, and you tune into the conversations. You become absorbed and settle into an easy chair where you listen, and listen and listen. The nurse talks of facing east, then of how to bring in a brother from Haiti, then of someone"s estranged father who has just been found and will be arriving soon, then of getting someone"s hair done before her son arrives, then of a prayer you had not heard of before, then of making sure a jug of water and a pan are available, then of how to change a diaper for someone"s mother and how to make it loving not shameful. You hear strains of a language you don"t understand and yet you do understand, and you hear tears and what seems to be poetry. Beads are chattering, someone tells another where to put the prayer mat, someone is singing gently – it seems to be a lullaby or maybe it's a psalm. A cry of pain triggers purposeful footsteps and soothing voices. A young man asks for a trundle bed next to his so his friend can stay over. You feel at home. You know everyone here belongs, feels welcome, wanted. Everyone is working.

As you rouse yourself from the moment of reverie you realise that you have experienced something extraordinary. Coming from the field of healthcare, as you do, you know that paradox; the paradox that says that dying well means living well – that also says that we are all different and yet all the same. And you know the reality that illness makes us all vulnerable in just the same way yet demands care that uses different approaches tailored to who is ill and who they are attached to. You know that it involves deep respect for the person and the perspective they bring. You know that you don't have to agree, but still you can respect and appreciate and learn and grow. But you wonder where the nurse learned to listen so well and to say the right things to such different people.

This modest volume gives the knowledge and the core skills set that can help you access that privileged state of connecting at such a deep level with people who were strangers before they arrived. It helps us ordinary healthcare people bring a little of the ideal into this imperfect world, and it helps us to participate in and share and pass on those moments of spiritual wealth.

Now in its third edition, this volume has continued to evolve, because we all do and the places we live always change. This edition is perfect for where we are now. May it change again and again in indefinite next editions so that it will always bring us what should be constant and unchanging: a tender respect for the human condition we live in and for the moments when we cease to live in the human condition and connect for the final moments of our present life with the existential.

Linda Emanuel
Director
Buehler Center on Aging
Northwestern University Chicago, USA
November 2003

Acknowledgements

The author and publishers would like to thank the following people for their valuable advice and critical comments on the manuscript while this book was being prepared:

For the first edition Mr AS Chhatwal, Editor of the *Sikh Courier*; Mrs Dana Banerjea of the National Association for the Welfare of Children in Hospital (NAWCH); Dr Z Badawi, Chairman of the Imams and Mosques Council; Sister Jotaka of the Amaravati Buddhist Centre; Mr Dennis Sibley of the then Buddhist Hospice Project, now the Buddhist Hospice Trust; Dharmadhara of Lessingham House, Norwich; Reverend Ian Ainsworth-Smith, Chaplain, St George's Hospital, London; and Saba Risalluddin of the Calamus Foundation.

Since the first edition many others have been extremely helpful in preparing the second and third editions of this book. Amongst them have been Professor Akbar Ahmed, for greater understanding of Islam; the Reverend Mark Cobb of Sheffield, for his inspiration in starting the Body and Soul Conferences; Naaz Coker, Chair of the Refugee Council, for general advice and particular help with Ismaili customs; Sister Harriet Copperman of the North London Hospice; the Right Reverend Richard Harries, Bishop of Oxford; the late Ernest Hochland of Haigh and Hochland Publications; Mei Sim Lai of Price Waterhouse, for her help with details about Chinese customs; the Reverend Eithne Lynch, Rector of Schull, West Cork; Vanessa Robshaw, for starting the Body and Soul Conferences and inviting me to participate; Rabbi Elaina Rothman of Cardiff Reform Synagogue; Deva Samaroo; Dennis Sibley of the Buddhist Hospice Trust; Michael Waterhouse, who was working on *Staying Close* as I was thinking about a third edition of this plus some other work; Canon John White of St George's House, Windsor; Rabbi Jonathan Wittenberg of the New North London Synagogue; the staff of the King's Fund Library for their patient chasing of references, and my family, for putting up endlessly with talk about caring for dying people of different faiths again.

This third edition is dedicated to the memory of the late Jim Rose, mentor and friend, whose work for the Runnymede Trust and whose seminal work on multi-ethnic Britain got me going on all this.

A note to the reader. Throughout this book we have used the female gender for nurses of both sexes and the male gender for patients of both sexes, unless specific examples require otherwise. The publishers and the author do not in any way wish to offend or discriminate against male nurses or female patients, but have chosen to use this convention to avoid the cumbersome use of both genders wherever a nurse or a patient is mentioned. We have chosen this convention because, at present, the majority of nurses in the UK are women.

1

Introduction to caring for dying people of different faiths

There is a real problem for many of us who are called upon to look after patients whose religion and customs are different from ours. It used to be easy. Britain was primarily a Christian society; in some ways it still is, but now many people in Britain are from totally different religious backgrounds, with quite different practices and beliefs. There are also many people who have no specific religion or religious and cultural tradition which might give them comfort, help and succour in the last days, weeks or months of their lives, or the lives of those they love. They are often the people who have most difficulty in knowing how to behave at the very end, for there is no very obvious ritual for them to follow, and that can be exacerbated for family and friends who are left behind if they too are not sure how to behave and what to do.

Finding out about the patient's beliefs

It is often tempting for carers, especially those with religious convictions, to assume that those who profess to a religion on a hospital form are in fact what they have stated, that is to say, for example, a practising and believing Muslim, Hindu or Jew. It cannot be stressed too often that this is no more likely to be true than if someone puts 'Church of England' down on the same form. It is quite likely to be merely a matter of labelling, of saying – in an increasingly diverse society that nevertheless recognises communities – that this is the community to which I belong.

Nevertheless, labels are important. It is not uncommon to find people who would describe themselves as agnostic Jews, Hindus or Muslims. This is because, for many people from the Indian sub-continent or those who have lived as minorities in Europe for centuries, the issue is not a straightforwardly religious one. It is to some extent anthropological; it is about ways of living lives, grouping ourselves within a community, marking the life-cycle occasions of births, marriages and deaths, and of distancing ourselves from other groups. Community is often defined by religious affiliation: one is a Muslim, Sikh, Hindu, Jew, Christian or whatever because of one's roots (very often because of one's name alone), regardless of beliefs or current religious practice. The distinguishing marks are often to do with what one eats and how one disposes of the dead and so on.

While the labels need to be respected, and food that is forbidden in one religion or another should not be served, it often requires a great deal more sensitivity than just reading the form to find out what the patient's religion is. Often the person concerned will volunteer information if asked in the right way: 'Well, you know, I'm not too bothered whether or not I see a priest ... I'm not really religious. Sometimes the family will make it very clear: 'Well, we're Jews, you know, but we don't practise much ... I shouldn't bother unduly'. The opposite may also manifest itself. The patient may become agitated and be comforted only by seeing a priest or by performing some ritual on his own in order to assuage some guilt or confusion. The family may tell the staff that the patient is deeply religious and often help the staff to provide the best possible care for the individual concerned. However, sometimes it turns out that it is the family that wants all the rituals, rather than the individual himself.

In all of these situations the burden on staff in the hospital, community or hospice is considerable. This has not been recognised until comparatively recently, because in a rather absurd way it was always believed that the hospital chaplain or the patient's own spiritual adviser could handle any problems. That time is now past. Hospital chaplains are often vastly over-burdened and cannot cope with all the cases they see. In the case of faiths other than Christianity, moreover, chaplains and official hospital visitors are often themselves very part-time. So nowadays carers themselves need the ability to handle such problems, in order to give proper and full care to seriously ill patients, for whom these religious and socio-religious concerns are of great importance.

Recognising the patient's needs

A great degree of comfort can be brought to a seriously ill or dying patient by the recognition of what their needs might possibly be. The fact that someone has bothered to ask whether it would be helpful to have a Bhagavad Gita or a pair of Jewish Sabbath candlesticks, or a Koran or a few drops of Ganges water brought in, makes all the difference to the individual who feels he is in unfamiliar surroundings and is often in pain or discomfort. Suddenly, here is someone who knows what might be required, who has taken the trouble to find out something about the individual patient's religion and culture, and who is offering to make special provision for the individual. It can make the difference between the patient regarding himself as just another person on the hospital conveyor belt or as someone whose individuality is being taken seriously. It can be enormously helpful, transforming the attitude of the patient concerned who may suddenly become more co-operative in treatment. The patient's relationship to the staff will also be enhanced with those who have shown such interest.

However, the converse can also be true. Some patients may describe themselves as Jews, Hindus or Muslims yet become quite angry when any offer of spiritual help is made. When nurses ask about their level of religious practice some patients may regard this as 'nosy and inquisitive'. The sensitivity required in this area is enormous; it is all too easy to upset a patient by forcing, or seeming to force, his own religion upon him. What has to be developed is a sensitivity towards the possible requirements of an individual patient, with some knowledge of the religious tradition from which he comes, rather than imposing an abandoned, half-forgotten, religious tradition upon him.

Recognising the different forms of each religion

Once a nurse has established that there is a need for, an interest in, or a willingness to find out what is available, she must be very careful to recognise all the different sects of every religion, for by no means all believers in a particular religion share the same degree of observance or the same theological beliefs. Indeed, many people who argue that they are from the same religion turn out to have less in common with each other than with people who hold the same intellectual position in other religious groupings. A classic example of this is the similarity, in some aspects, between Christian fundamentalists, the people who believe that there is no human element in the story of the Gospels and who argue for a strong belief in Hell, and orthodox Jews who believe quite literally that God gave the Torah, the Five Books of Moses, to Moses on Mount Sinai. Those intellectual positions, undoubting and uncritical, have in some ways more in common with each other than either does with the more liberal view in their own religion.

In most, but not all, religions, there is an orthodox and a progressive or liberal wing. There are also variations in types of the religion, as distinct from intellectual position, often due to the country or area of origin. Thus there are Shi'ite and Sunni Muslims, Ismaili Muslims, followers of the Aga Khan, as well as Ahmaddiya who are a rather different group. There are Sephardi and Ashkenazi Jews, who may be orthodox, conservative, reform or liberal by grouping. There are Roman Catholics and various types of Christians from the Protestant traditions, from the established to the free churches. There are Hindus of a wide variety of beliefs and there are more and less fundamentalist Sikhs. There are Chinese Christians and Chinese Buddhists, who nevertheless share a great deal in respect for ancestors, and there are Shintoists and Buddhists from Japan, again linked by ancestor respect.

All these variations and shades of view need to be borne in mind by anyone caring for people belonging to religious, cultural and ethnic groups with which the nurse is less than familiar. However, it is not all that difficult. The truth of the matter is that usually the patient or the patient's family is so delighted that any interest is being taken in their religious or cultural life that they will pour out information and detail, and in fact leave the nurse who asked the original question feeling that she has opened up an important and sensitive area. Nurses can learn much from this experience. It can also be immensely exciting. Nevertheless, before the learning process can begin properly, it is as well to have in mind where the main differences in attitudes tend to lie.

Areas for examination

The first requirement for anyone caring for a patient and wishing to recognise his spiritual and cultural needs is to know something of the basic beliefs of the religion concerned. In each of the succeeding chapters, a very brief and therefore necessarily simplistic summary of beliefs has been given. These range from belief in God or gods to concepts of the afterlife and immortality of the soul, from the nature of human life to the idea of sacred texts. When dealing with the dying patient, it is very important to have some idea of his beliefs about immortality of the soul and the afterlife – for obvious reasons. However, those are not the only areas of interest and a more general knowledge can be very helpful.

One basic and practical consideration is whether there are last rites – whether there are rules about who can touch the body, questions about confession, about prayers, about leaving the dead person alone and so on. These are listed in no specific order, just as they occur in the course of the nurse's duties. One of the reasons for writing the first edition of this book nearly 20 years ago was to try and order the thinking about these issues, and to see how prohibitions and taboos in various religions link in with the basic structure of their beliefs. For instance, it is impossible to understand laws and prohibitions about not leaving human bodies alone after death without having some idea of what that particular religion or philosophy has to say about the nature of human life and its value. Without that, the most common response is for the nurse to try to impose her own views – for want of anything 'better' to do. This is rarely done out of arrogance or a desire to effect a bedside conversion, but merely out of a lack of understanding and sympathy.

In each case, questions need to be asked about the value of human life. These need to be expanded into questions about the nature of human life in the here and now, as against any future life or spiritual immortality. Then there is the whole area of what it is permissible to do with or to the body – what parts can be replaced in transplants or whether that has any effect on the nature of individual immortality. What is the attitude to pain relieving drugs which can, arguably, shorten life? How firmly held are beliefs in this area? The questions are endless and by no means easy to answer, but a nurse who wants to give comprehensive care to patients who hold views different from her own at least needs to grapple with the questions, even if she does not know the answers. More than that, she needs to think out her own views on these subjects, because only with a secure basis to one's own thinking can one really learn and understand other people's.

Once attitudes to human life itself have been thought out, other issues have to be considered. For instance, what does that particular religion say about last rites? Some religious groupings, notably Roman Catholics, regard them as essential. In others, there are no such things. In some religions, it would be normal and right for a person to be told if he were dying, if he did not already know. In others, this would be anathema, for he might then not make the effort at recovery and lose the will to fight which might give him a little longer of this life here on earth.

All these are issues which need to be explored, for they may materially affect the way the patient is treated. They may also help the nurse to understand the patient she is caring for in the last stages of life. Many people have a real need for spiritual care and comfort in these last stages, but they are not always available from chaplains and visitors, nor indeed are these always the only appropriate people to give them.

Obviously, we are dealing here with some fundamental questions about the nature of nursing, and the extent to which nursing care covers the spiritual aspect of life. Twenty years ago this was a subject barely touched upon in nursing training and education, or in debates about what was properly part of nursing care. Now, however, books are written, articles published in learned and professional journals, conferences are over-subscribed and short courses over-booked, such is the interest in spiritual care in nursing, long overdue though it is. Nevertheless, for practical purposes, all nurses need some basic knowledge and the life, in those last days, weeks and months, of many dying patients will be immeasurably improved if nurses have some awareness of their spiritual needs, and try, very unobtrusively, to minister to them.

Two last points need to be made.

- Nurses themselves should not underestimate just how stressful dealing with dying patients and their families can be. It can often make the whole process much easier if the nurse herself knows something of what the expectations of the patient and the family are likely to be.
- This book is just a beginning; it tries to set some of the boundaries and to introduce the caring nurse to some of the philosophies, religions and ways of life her patients may have.

Anyone who wants a thorough knowledge of the subject or subjects, however, would be well advised to read, study and discuss these issues in greater depth, and some titles which might be helpful can be found in the bibliography at the end of this book.

2

Judaism

Story of the Jewish people and their faith

Judaism is a religion largely of a people, the Jews. Whilst by no means distinguishable by ethnicity (there are black, brown and white Jews of a variety of different racial types), there is a strong sense of people-hood amongst the Jews and a sense of group loyalty and support for each other. The old adage used to be that Jews 'looked after their own' but, although that is true in some circumstances, it is by no means universal and Jews suffer a great deal from the fragmentation of families found throughout British society.

Jews regard Abraham as the founder of Judaism. In terms of the Bible stories, Abraham was the first of the three patriarchs who together are regarded as the founding fathers of the people of Israel. Jacob, Abraham's grandson, had the name Israel conferred upon him and his descendants at the end of a night-long struggle with a mysterious stranger. According to the Bible, the two wrestled until dawn. The stranger then asked to be released. Jacob refused to do so without a blessing. The stranger asked his name and, when told, said:

You shall no longer be called Jacob, but Israel, for you have striven with God and with Man and have prevailed.

The name 'Israel' that attaches to the Jewish people and later to the Jewish state means 'one who wrestles with God'.

The history of Judaism is more complicated, however. Whatever the historical truth of the journey from Ur of the Chaldees to the land of Canaan, with Abraham following a divine call, Judaism as a religion regards itself as the product of two journeys. The first is Abraham's, with Lot, of the early stories in the book of Genesis. They went from Mesopotamia to the land of Canaan and Abraham settled there and made it his tribal home. Then, three generations later, there was a famine in the land and they journeyed to Egypt to get food, where they encountered Joseph who had been sold into slavery by his brothers who could neither stand his arrogance nor their father's favouritism towards him. Joseph became vizier to one of the Pharaohs and was in charge of food supplies. He recognised his brothers and eventually invited them all down to Egypt, where they lived happily for some time. Then there came a Pharaoh 'who knew not Joseph' and who started treating the Israelites as slaves. From that point, things became worse and worse until, led by Moses, they left Egypt (the Exodus) and journeyed for 40 years in the wilderness before reaching the promised land.

To what extent this is actually true, in that it can be proved historically, is a matter of considerable debate. What can be said, however, is that the folk memory of journeying from slavery to freedom became one of the most important motifs in Jewish thought. The reminders are constant – in one version of the Ten Commandments, for instance, the reason for observing the Sabbath is given as having been slaves in Egypt. The implications are twofold: firstly, that you know what it is to have no rest, and secondly, that you should give your servants and animals rest, precisely because you know what it is to be a slave.

Because this is such a strong motif in Judaism, the Egypt experience, as one might describe it, figures large. The Sabbath, for those who are religious, is of great importance. The festival of Passover, despite not being as important a festival as the New Year and the Day of Atonement (jointly termed the High Holy Days), is of great sentimental and emotional value to even the most disaffected Jews. They regard themselves as if they had been there, as if they had been freed from Egyptian slavery.

During the journey through the wilderness, the children of Israel were given the Torah or the Pentateuch and became governed by the rule of law. Orthodox Jews believe that the Torah was handed down literally by God to Moses on Mount Sinai. Progressive (conservative, reform and liberal) Jews believe that it was divinely inspired, but written down by human beings at different times, and that there are contradictions within it and elements which are human rather than divine. The extent to which Jews stick to the letter of the law varies considerably. Their degree of adherence to Jewish law can only be found out by asking them.

Though practice varies, most Jews, however unobservant, would understand the expression 'performing a mitzvah'. Literally this means performing a commandment, but has come to mean doing a good turn. Jews who hold no religious beliefs themselves would often feel sufficiently Jewish to be offended by crucifixes hung all over the walls, or by being asked to kneel for prayers which Jews never do.

It is worth mentioning perhaps that even for the least religious Jew there is a strong sense of the value of being human, and therefore of human life. It derives from a religious belief – that God created human beings in His own image. However, it has extended well beyond the strictly religious sphere and means that doctors and other healthcare workers are always immensely respected by Jews as those who preserve and cherish human life. Because of that attitude to human life, all positive religious laws can be broken (not the negative ones, like the prohibition on murder) in order to save or preserve human life. Thus, no Jew has to observe festivals and the Sabbath when terminally ill. Nevertheless, as with people of other faiths and cultures, many will choose to do so.

The Sabbath and Passover

However orthodox or liberal Jews happen to be, there are some things most would undeniably find comforting, unless they do not practise their Judaism at all. Such things include candles being lit for them on a Friday night at the beginning of the

Sabbath (the Jewish Sabbath runs from sundown on Friday to sundown on Saturday), being given unleavened bread at Passover (called matzah and available almost everywhere throughout the country), and even a visit from a rabbi at Passover. This visit would be bringing no last rites, which Judaism does not have, but instead some symbols from the Passover table: the bitter herbs representing the bitterness of the slavery in Egypt, and the sweet paste of apples, nuts, cinnamon and wine representing the mortar they used as slaves to stick the bricks together for the Pharaoh's store-cities – it also takes away the taste of the bitter herbs!

Food restrictions

There are innumerable things which the Jewish patient would find helpful from staff. The orthodox Jew adheres to the dietary laws very strictly and will only eat meat which is kosher (fit). That has to be arranged with the kosher meals service and is no problem. Often more difficult is the less orthodox patient who keeps some, but not all, of the laws. For instance, he might well not eat the forbidden foods, such as pork and shellfish, but might eat meat slaughtered in the normal way provided it came from a permitted animal. He might also have qualms about mixing milk and meat at the same meal, due to an original prohibition of 'seething the kid in its mother's milk'; he might require quite a time, up to six hours, after eating a meat product or meat meal before he would consume anything with milk in it. In all these cases, it is best for the nurse to ask the patient or the patient's family, assuming that she has some awareness that there are food restrictions and a glimmering of an idea in which direction these might lie.

Food is immensely important in Jewish life and it may seem, to many people who are not Jewish, to be a cause for quite unreasonable concern. In the case of very ill and dying patients, it will not be unusual for the family to be more concerned about an unwillingness or inability to eat than about anything else. Indeed, favoured delicacies may be brought in and the time-honoured cure-all (in European Jewry) of chicken soup may well be tried. Amusing though this might seem, it is a sign of a very deep, strong hold on life. For in Judaism it is *this* life which is of importance, *this* world and all it has to offer. Eating is a sign of a hold on this world. Of all the religions, Judaism could perhaps legitimately be described as the most 'this life' affirming. Although orthodox Jews say every morning that they believe in an afterlife and, indeed, in physical resurrection of the dead, the ideas surrounding this whole area are hazy and uncertain, and there is huge variety in the actual belief held. What is certain is what happens in the here and now, and it is about the here and now that human beings should really concern themselves.

Attitude towards death

This grip on life often makes Jews less than good at dealing with dying patients. Strangely, it is not the uncertainty about the after-life which causes the problem, but the emphasis put on the here and now – for the person who is dying is plainly not going to be around in the here and now for much longer, and is therefore, in some strange way, no longer worthy of consideration. Although Judaism is extremely good at looking after the bereaved and gives them support and comfort, the dying person is often neglected and brought little in the way of comfort. Recently, the Jewish community has become more aware of this lack and tries to work more with those who are dying and their families, offering some Jewish social care if appropriate. The Jewish community is deeply involved in the North London hospice, the first truly multi-faith, as opposed to non-denominational, hospice in the UK. However, attitudes to how to cope with dying vary, of course, and there are strict laws about not short-ening a dying person's life, which imply that it is considered of immense value. The only thing that is permitted in strict Jewish law is the stopping of some external factor, such as a terrible noise, which is preventing the person from dying.

Often a dying Jew does ask to see a rabbi. There are no last rites in Judaism and a visit from the rabbi is not essential. However, if a rabbi is asked for, the nurse should ask whether the family is orthodox and when the orthodox rabbi should be called, or whether they are reform or liberal and when a reform or liberal rabbi should be called. Often, if it really is near the end, the rabbi will say some prayers with the patient and try to get him to say the first line of a prayer called the Shema:

Hear O Israel, the Lord is our God, the Lord is one.

There is the chance too for a private confession – not out loud to the rabbi – and the last words the patient speaks might well be that line of prayer. Very often, the family is much comforted by the presence of a rabbi, partly because it seems appropriate, but partly also because there are many things to be done at the time of a death and they want to make sure that they have got it right.

What to do with the body

Traditionally, when a Jew dies, the body is left for about eight minutes while a feather is left over the mouth and nostrils and watched for signs of breathing. If there are no such signs, then the eyes and mouth are gently closed by the son or nearest relative. That having been done, the arms are extended down the sides of the body, and the lower jaw is bound up before rigor mortis sets in. Then, again traditionally, the body is placed on the floor with feet towards the door, covered with a sheet and a lighted candle is placed just by the head. If it is the Sabbath or a festival, the body cannot be moved, though the chin can be bound up. However, in most hospitals and hospices it would be impossible to leave a dead person in the ward for that long so, unless the person died in a side ward which is not needed immediately, it is best to move the body to a room where it can remain until the sexton comes to remove it.

  All these first acts of shutting the eyes and laying the arms straight are traditionally done by members of the family or by other fellow Jews. If someone dies in a hospital or nursing home some way away from his nearest relative, this may not be possible. It is then perfectly permissible, even for the strictest of orthodox Jews, for a member of staff to perform these first acts, but what is not allowed is for the body to be moved and left on its own. A series of guidelines issued in 1960 by the Sexton's office of the United Synagogue Burial Society says the following:

> *Where it is not possible to obtain the services of a Jewish chaplain, it is permissible for hospital staff to carry out the following: Close the eyes. Tie up the jaw. Keep arms and hands straight and by the sides of the body. Any tubes or instruments in the body should be removed and the incision plugged. The corpse should then be wrapped in a plain sheet without religious emblems, and placed in the mortuary or other special room for Jewish bodies.*

Once the initial limb-straightening is carried out, the body is not left alone. Orthodox Jews and some non-orthodox ones continue the custom of having watchers, who stay with the body day and night and recite Psalms all the time. That time is not usually very long, since Jews are commanded to bury their dead as quickly as possible. This too tends to be preserved as a tradition even by non-observant Jews, and the lengthy delay between death and funeral quite common in other cultures is virtually unheard of amongst Jews. Delays can and do occur of course, particularly in the case of post-mortem examinations. These are often resisted by orthodox Jews (they are forbidden unless ordered by the civil authorities) and the giving of organs for transplant use, with the exception of corneas, is also frowned on in most cases. Reform, liberal and non-observant Jews do not share these feelings about post-mortems, where they are for the benefit of future generations of human beings, nor on the whole do they object to the donation of organs for transplant. Many will carry donor cards, but it is certainly worth asking the families of non-observant and progressive Jews if they are prepared to give the organs of the dead person for this purpose.

Jewish funerals

Once the immediate formalities are completed, the funeral has to be arranged. The family normally does this, but in a few cases, where there is no family, the solicitor or the hospital social worker has to make the arrangements. If the dead person was an orthodox Jew, then burial is the only option, in a Jewish cemetery. If he was a progressive Jew, or totally non-observant, then cremation is also a possibility. However, if the staff who have to make the arrangements are not certain which is preferred by the person concerned, then the safer option is to choose burial as this is still considerably more common amongst Jews. Many people argue, orthodox or not, that the burial, and the casting of shovels full of earth on the coffin by the mourners themselves, has a very powerful and salutary effect – it brings home the reality, but it also allows them to feel that they themselves have buried their dead. If the person was orthodox, then the body will be removed and all washing will be done by a group called the chevra kaddisha, the holy assembly, who carry out ritual purification of the dead and for whom the last attentions to the dead are a great religious duty and honour. Most non-orthodox Jews do not have this ritual purification and the body is treated in the normal way, but a few do. Once again, where possible, family and friends should be asked what would be fitting.

After the funeral has taken place, there is a formal period of mourning, for seven days initially, when the bereaved stay at home to receive visitors and sit on low chairs. It is a time when evening prayers are held in the home and friends, relatives, and members of the community come to pay their respects and to show their sympathy and support. For many people this is a very comforting experience. They find the constant company of people ready to listen to their agony very helpful. It is clear that this ritual is of considerable value psychologically, for it encourages people to express their grief and their friends to listen to and understand it. Their first meal at the beginning of the seven-day period, known as the shiva (which means seven), is a traditional mourners' meal brought to them by friends. It consists of hard boiled eggs and beigels (round rolls) and, in some communities, lentils. All these are seen as round foods, symbolising the cycle of life and death. Other rituals, such as the cutting of clothes before the funeral and not shaving or cutting the nails, are also seen as comforting – a way of marking a terrible loss, with outward signs that people will recognise, and imposing a duty on others to come to the mourners' house for prayers. The shiva is the first part of 30 days of full mourning, succeeded by 11 months before the first anniversary. The tombstone is usually consecrated just before the year is up, to mark the end of formal mourning. The anniversary – yahrzeit – is marked with prayers and the lighting of a special yahrzeit candle, whilst those who were bereaved are themselves still alive.

Jews have such different views about the afterlife that this subject is not something in which staff would want to get involved. The ritual of support for mourners is, however, universal amongst Jews, although not always formalised in the seven-day pattern of the shiva. Dying Jews and their families often find it helpful to think of the support of the mourners, and the strong emphasis on the living. It is also often a last wish of a dying Jew that someone should say kaddish, the mourner's prayer, for him. It can be a source of considerable comfort to a Jew to know that the staff, if no family is available, know roughly what to do and will make the necessary arrangements. It can also be a comfort to know that someone will make sure that kaddish is said when the person goes to join his ancestors – for the bond of saying kaddish is one that unites generations of Jews in a powerful and important way. This is clear during the memorial service on the holiest day of the year, the Day of Atonement, when everyone remembers and thinks of their dear departed, and says kaddish for them, as the emotion rises within the synagogue.

3

Christianity

Many readers of this book may have had a Christian upbringing – perhaps the bulk of readers – or have lived in the UK or other countries where Christianity is still dominant in the culture if not in practice. For those readers for whom this is true, they are asked to forgive the author for the degree of ignorance assumed in the writing of this chapter. It seemed more sensible to treat Christianity, like the other religions, as something that a considerable proportion of readers would know little about.

History and faith

Christianity is the religion of the followers of Jesus, whom they proclaim to be the Son of God and through whom they approach God himself. The extent to which Jesus is viewed as part of the godhead varies according to which branch of Christianity is under consideration. Most tenets of the faith are the same, whichever group is being examined, but the emphasis sometimes varies, as for instance with the concept of the virgin birth; some sections of Christianity are emphatic about it, while others are less dogmatic about its literal truth.

The fundamental belief of Christianity dates back to Jesus, born in Bethlehem some 2000 years ago. He was born into a Jewish family and community and fitted into a school of charismatic teaching and miracle working of contemporary Galilee. He taught and performed his miracles mainly during the last three years of his life, in areas which are now part of modern Israel, Jordan and Syria. The country was then under Roman rule, under the governor Pontius Pilate.

His followers believed Jesus to be the Messiah, the anointed one, saviour of the Jews. The word in Greek for Messiah is *Khristos*, meaning anointed one, hence the names Christ and Christian. Jesus was an extremely successful and charismatic figure and attracted a large following. In itself, that inspired jealousy in some who felt threatened by his popularity. They, along with the Roman rulers of the time, wanted to overthrow him and so in approximately 33 AD Jesus was crucified just outside Jerusalem.

The beliefs of Christianity can be summed up in the Apostle's creed:

I believe in God the Father Almighty, Creator of Heaven and earth; and in Jesus Christ his only Son, Our Lord, who was conceived by the Holy Spirit, born of the Virgin Mary; suffered under Pontius Pilate, was crucified, dead and buried, he descended into hell; on the third day he rose again from the dead, he ascended into heaven; is seated at the right hand of God the Father Almighty; from hence he shall come to judge the quick and the dead. I believe in the Holy Ghost, the holy Catholic Church, the Communion of Saints, the forgiveness of sins, the resurrection of the body, and the life of the world to come. Amen.

Christians believe in following the example of Jesus and that that way lies the salvation of humanity. Jesus is the human embodiment of a loving, just and personal God; he lived as a man and was crucified for the sins of humanity, but he was resurrected from the grave and ascended into heaven to sit at the hand of God.

The festivals of Christianity

Christmas and Easter are the best known and most universally observed of the Christian festivals. Christmas has become very secularised in the UK and elsewhere in the world, with massive

commercial exploitation and relatively little religious significance. Nevertheless, it should have considerable religious significance in celebrating the birth of Jesus; some of the most beautiful
church services and music are designed for Christmas Eve and
Christmas Day.

Lent lasts for 40 days, beginning on Ash Wednesday and
ending on Good Friday. It commemorates Jesus spending 40
days in the desert. It is used as a time for reflection, when many
Christians do without one pleasure or another (e.g. food, alcohol,
smoking) and try to be better people. Christians may well use
Lent as a period for self-analysis and reassessment; those who
are terminally ill may use Lent to prepare themselves for the end
and to be better able to deal with their own deaths.

Good Friday marks the end of Lent. It is a solemn day in the
Church, for it marks the day of Christ's crucifixion. The date
varies (Easter is calculated according to the lunar calendar but is
different in the Orthodox Church from the Roman Catholic and
Protestant churches) but is some time in March or April. Good
Friday used to be a day of long church sermons and solemn
behaviour. To some extent it still is, although the tradition of
lengthy preaching is dying out in all the churches.

Easter Day is the celebration of Christ's resurrection from the
dead and is usually a day of reflection and great joy. It is seen
by many Christians as the most important festival of the religious calendar. Many Christians who are not regular churchgoers would nonetheless tend to want to attend church on Good
Friday and Easter Day.

There is also the popular custom of the giving of chocolate
eggs. These are not necessarily connected with Christian symbol-
ism, though eggs as a symbol of spring, new life and rebirth are
elements of many religions' spring festivals. Different traditions
have their own customs. Some blow real eggs and paint the
shells in bright colours. Others have chocolate eggs. Still others
eat hard boiled eggs which have been brightly painted. The eggs
are accompanied with other special foods, notably Easter cakes
of one sort or another, often with a dairy product content such
as cheesecake or the Russian pashka.

Whitsun is the last of the Christian festivals. It occurs 50 days
(hence PENTECOST, as *pentkoste* is Greek for 50th) after Easter,

corresponding with the Jewish Pentecost. Its message is that during the festival of Pentecost the Holy Spirit came amongst Christ's disciples after his death and enabled them to talk to and converse with members of the crowds in a variety of different languages. Particular importance is attached to the experience of the Pentecost by Christians of all denominations in the charismatic tradition. This lays special emphasis on the gifts of the spirit which may include speaking in tongues – a relatively important part of the belief and practice of charismatic and some black and African churches, formerly somewhat disapproved of by other adherents to the Christian faith.

Beliefs

Christians of virtually all denominations believe in an afterlife. Concepts of this afterlife range from a liberal view of some kind of quite different existence of the soul in a world to come to a fairly fundamentalist view of Heaven and Hell.

The people who follow Jesus' example in this life will go to Heaven, which will be a perfect existence, and Hell, a place of torment, is the alternative. Beliefs about the exact nature of Heaven and Hell vary considerably between individuals as well as from group to group. For most western Christians, Heaven and Hell are viewed more as concepts than as statements of literal truth. Underlying all the varying theologies, however, is the view that a new spiritual birth takes place by accepting Jesus into one's life. Some Christian groups proselytise actively in order to save the souls of as many unbelievers as possible. Others, while believing that salvation comes through an acceptance of the Christian message, believe it wrong to proselytise, regarding religious belief as a matter of personal choice for the individual. There are also a few very liberal Christian groups who believe that those who adhere to other faiths have found their own way to God, and that it would be wrong to suggest to them that Christianity is in any way superior. Christians view impending death as a time of looking towards the afterlife. Those who feel reasonably satisfied with the way in which they have lived – and there is a considerable amount of self-

assessment amongst people of all religions when nearing death –
approach their death with some degree of equanimity, believing
that Christians share the hope of a new life beyond death.
Others, especially if they view illness and death as a punishment
from God, may experience feelings of intense anger and disillu-
sionment with God. It is frequently very helpful for people in
this position to explore these feelings rather than to suppress
them. For them, a visit from a sympathetic hospital chaplain or
minister can be very helpful. These feelings are frequently shared
by relatives and friends of the dying person. Some lapsed Christians may discover a renewed faith and trust in God through
pastoral visits.

   What is very obvious, as pointed out by the Bishop of Oxford,
the Rt Reverend Richard Harries, on many occasions, is the
contrast between the attitudes to death one encounters amongst
Anglicans in the 20th and 21st century and those held by people
in the 17th century, and, of course, much earlier. The sense of
judgement after death is fading, even amongst those who are
communicants, even amongst those who regard themselves as
fairly traditional, if not orthodox, in their beliefs. The emphasis
has come to be much more on this world, even though the same
theologians who encourage people to have concern for the poor
and disadvantaged in this world also ask Christians to have
hope in the face of death. However, if final judgement, if Heaven
and Hell, are so unreal to modern Anglicans, why should one
worry about hope or faith at the point of death? Modern Christians are rediscovering a sense of the rightness of dying well,
dying by giving all they are back to God to be refashioned and
used according to His desires. That is the modern Anglican sense
that is beginning to be real – a sense of giving oneself back to the
creator, having lived (if one can) a good life, or as good as
possible, and died a good, resolved death. Much of this has been
influenced by Freud. Much has also been influenced by the
experience of the First World War which destroyed so much of
Britain's youth – how could they be facing eternal judgement?
The Christian faith asks people to give themselves back, a
consciously willed love of God and humanity. That is a modern
form of Christian attitude to death and it is that sense of giving
oneself back that is enormously important to many believing

Christians – a sense nurses need to look out for as people are readying themselves for what they see as some kind of final sacrifice.

One last point: Christianity has, at some points in its history, had an ambivalent or even negative attitude to the human body. It has been regarded as dirty, unnecessary, merely the vessel for the soul, and worthy of affliction in order to acquire spiritual refinement or wholeness. However, this needs to be set against a traditional belief in physical resurrection, as promised by Jesus' resurrection. Added to that is a traditional Christian antipathy to cremation – much diluted in modern western societies – because of the difficulty with physical resurrection from ashes. However, for most people, as Michael Waterhouse points out in his elegant book, *Staying Close*, the reflection in the mirror is the nature of the self – we cannot imagine ourselves without our bodies. Our concept of soul or spirit tends to be very physical and that is not helped by concepts of Paradise – amid trees, flowers, gardens (*pairadaeza* is Old Persian for royal park or garden) – and the Garden of Eden. Add to these the Elysian Fields of Greek myth, the Happy Fields of ancient Egypt and the Fields of Heaven for Tibetan Buddhists, and the fact that Christians have a sense of the body being pre-eminent over the spirit or soul is not unique. The sense of self in western countries is well developed and strongly linked to the body, a fact nurses need to be aware of when tending people who are Christians, or who come from that religion, as they watch their bodies disintegrate as they prepare for death.

Different branches of Christianity

Christianity is divided into many groups. Because they behave differently at the time of death, it is worth describing the groups briefly. The three main groups are the Roman Catholic Church, the Protestant churches and the eastern Orthodox churches. When facing death and bereavement, people's cultural background may have as important an effect on behaviour as their religious background. The Orthodox Church developed in the 6th century AD when the Church in Eastern Europe and Asia

Minor took a different path in matters of doctrine and practice from the Roman Catholic Church in the West.

The Orthodox Church

Orthodox patients may request a Bible, a crucifix and a prayer book. Some may bring in a small family icon. Nurses may need to exercise some degree of tact if the icon is a particularly valuable work of art and may need to encourage patients or their families to consider appropriate insurance cover. Indeed, nurses may find themselves discouraging the patient from keeping the icon in hospital, for this practical reason. The easiest thing is to encourage the family, if available, to bring the icon in and out when they visit. For many orthodox patients an icon brings great comfort, so that discouraging its presence in hospital is a difficult thing to do. Nurses need to be sensitive to the importance of the presence of the icon in each individual case.

Last rites and burial

Orthodox Christians are usually buried, but there is often a formal lying-in-state in the church, in the coffin, so that family and friends can come and pay their last respects. Before death, the local Orthodox priest should be asked to visit the patient. The patient's family and friends could be encouraged to organise the visit. In most cases, the priest will hear the last confession, anoint the patient with the oil of the sick and give communion. Many Orthodox Christians attach considerable importance to this event. Once this has taken place it becomes much easier to help them. An Orthodox patient can be laid out as normal. There are no restrictions about handling the body.

The Roman Catholic Church

Roman Catholics believe that the Pope is the spiritual successor to Saint Peter and that he is invested with Christ's authority. The Roman Catholic Church has a formal hierarchy of bishops and priests which is focused on the Vatican in Rome. There are many religious orders for men and women, some of whom are involved in nursing and caring. Roman Catholics are often regular churchgoers and communicants if they practise their religion at all, though in recent years a considerable falling-off in practice has taken place in Western Europe particularly, including in Ireland, Italy and Spain. Services at the bedside may be very important to Roman Catholics, and the parish priest or the Roman Catholic hospital chaplain should be called in.

Last rites and burial

If the patient's condition requires that they take nil by mouth, nurses will need to be sensitive to the needs of a Roman Catholic patient to receive Holy Communion. When the patient is actually dying, the priest will normally minister the sacrament of the sick which is popularly called the last rites. The priest anoints the patient with oil and prays for God to ease the patient's suffering and administers absolution, a statement of God's forgiveness for the patient's past sins.

The patient may already have requested a copy of the Bible or a Catholic prayer book. A rosary, medallions of the Pope, Saints, or the Virgin Mary, and often a crucifix may be brought by the patient's family and friends. The Virgin Mary is of great importance in Roman Catholicism – Catholics frequently pray through her and ask her for mediation. Occasionally patients will keep holy water from Lourdes by their beds, or from other shrines thought to be places of miraculous cures. When a Catholic patient dies, having received the sacrament of the sick, the family may ask for the patient's hands to be placed in an attitude of prayer holding a crucifix or rosary. In all other ways, laying out can proceed as normal.

Great emphasis may be put on the funeral and this is particularly the case if the family is Irish in origin, when the funeral may take place very quickly after the death. It is usually a burial – and a requiem mass will very likely be of huge importance. Requiem masses, so called because of the words of the Introit – 'Requiem aeternam dona eis, Domine' ('Give them eternal peace, O Lord') – are sung traditionally in plainsong, but have many wonderful settings by most of the major composers, e.g. Mozart, Berlioz, Fauré and Verdi. Such masses are often the funeral service themselves – a mass changed for the purposes of the burial. The knowledge that a proper funeral with a requiem mass will be said, or sung, can be of great comfort to someone dying who is a Catholic by upbringing or belief. If they are Irish in origin, they may also want reassurance that there will be a wake afterwards, with cake, sandwiches, drink and a long night of commiseration – a kind of party for the dead person and the bereaved.

The Protestant churches

Protestant Christianity developed during the 16th century as a reaction to what were perceived as the worst excesses and abuses of the Catholic Church at the time. The Church of England, while it adheres to the principles of the Reformation, maintains the traditional order of bishops and priests also associated with the Roman Catholic and Orthodox churches. The Free Churches and the Church of Scotland maintain a variety of practices which may differ in some respects from that of the Church of England and nurses will need to establish to which Christian tradition a patient belongs. A number (around 300) of Church of England chaplains are employed full time by the National Health Service (NHS) in hospitals, although licensed by the bishop of the diocese. There are also usually some part-time Roman Catholic and Free Church chaplains. In recent years, the chaplains' approach has tended to be far more ecumenical. There has been a real improvement in pastoral care in hospitals as a result of the ecumenical approach gaining so much ground. Non-believers or those who are only nominally Christian have frequently welcomed visits from the chaplain on a social basis, although the patient's wishes should always be respected.

Practices

The traditional Christian sacraments of baptism, confession, Holy Communion, laying on of hands and anointing are usually available if required. Hospital chaplains can provide all of these and

Communion can be brought to a ward *for* an individual or a group. In the Protestant tradition, there are fewer formally observed last rites, although many practising Anglican patients may wish to receive the sacrament of the sick. Some patients ask for Holy Communion and others prefer someone to be with them. It is also often very helpful to the family if a chaplain is present.

The Religious Society of Friends (Quakers) has no clergy, but the overseer from a local Friends Meeting House can be helpful. Often all that is required is the presence of another Quaker, and the ministry of the hospital chaplain is usually quite acceptable.

Practices may vary in groups such as the Plymouth Brethren and also with other religious groups not formally Christian, including Jehovah's Witnesses and Mormons. The best advice in these circumstances is to ask the patient or the family.

The variety of belief amongst Christians is considerable and often the best way to find out about beliefs and practices is to ask the patient or his family. However, belief in an afterlife and a sense of being united with relatives or friends after death and of experiencing a fuller relationship with God may help to ease the pain of accepting the impending death. It can be helpful for nurses to be aware of this.

It is also easier for nurses to care for Christian patients with the support of the permanent full- or part-time presence of a chaplain. He or she can be very helpful and supportive to patients, relatives and staff. Hospital chaplains are trained to provide comfort to the very ill and dying. Nevertheless, nurses can still find themselves on the ward in the middle of the night on their own, facing difficult and agonising spiritual questions from their patients. In these circumstances most chaplains are happy to be called out or consulted, although there are times when that is not possible.

Advice will always be given by the Hospital Chaplaincies Council at Church House, Great Smith Street, Westminster, London SW1P 3NZ; tel: 020 7898 1894; fax: 020 7898 1891. This is an ecumenical body on which the main Christian denominations are represented.

4

African and Afro-Caribbean beliefs and customs

There are large numbers of people of Afro-Caribbean origins or African origins in the UK and their customs are often very similar to those of other Christians or Muslims, but, particularly in the case of Christians, with some notable exceptions.

Beliefs

The spirit life is much more real and live to many Afro-Caribbean people. In some cases, there will be a second funeral after the first one when the body is buried, in which the hovering spirits, around after a death, are laid to rest so that they cannot disturb the living. This has to be seen alongside a real belief in spirits which inhabit people, and the use of exorcism as a way of dealing with evil spirits inhabiting the living.

This is not, as often seen by other Christians with western origins, some form of primitive belief – though sometimes it appears that way, particularly when children are subjected to exorcism to get rid of their evil spirits. Instead, it is more like the belief in spirits and the presence of ancestors to be found in Chinese and Japanese beliefs. The ancestors are ever present and the spirits of the dead take a close interest in the family and business affairs of the living.

All this is complicated because of the rise of new religious groupings and particular local customs which depend on the country or region of origin. Caring staff should ask for information which might help them care better for someone from a specific African grouping, but meanwhile should be aware that Christianity or Islam will be the most likely faiths, with some variations as to local custom.

There are two exceptions worth mentioning: Rastafarians and African believers in evil spirits. The first, Rastafarians, are a considerable grouping in the UK. Recognised normally by their dreadlocks (uncut, washed and plaited hair), they follow the Nazirite vow of separation which forbids certain foods and activities, including contact with dead bodies. This makes them similar to the priestly group amongst the Jewish population, who also – and for some of the same reasons – do not go anywhere near a dead body. The founder of Rastafarianism in Jamaica in the 1920s, Marcus Garvey, viewed his people as a form of priesthood – hence the vow – and encouraged them to behave in a priestly, dignified and classically African way. The theory is that Rastafarianism is the religion of ancient Ethiopia, and the hats Rastafarians wear are red, green and gold, the colours of Ethiopia.

The other difference, difficult to cope with but essential to understand, is the belief amongst many Africans, including many African Christians, in evil spirits which are sent by someone to do harm. Thus a person dying an untimely death is often thought to have been harmed by the evil spirit sent by an enemy – or a woman who is childless is seen as having her life channels blocked by evil spirits, again possibly sent by someone. Spirits are very present as ancestors, who are thought to carry on the same activities as those who are still alive, but the belief in evil spirits, and forms of magic, is somewhat different. Since this belief is widespread in some African communities, it may be the case that the person who is identified (perhaps through prayer, perhaps through a witch doctor) as having sent the evil spirit has to make some kind of recompense as a form of acknowledgement, even though this probably has no effect on the disease. The result of this is usually some monetary payment from one person to the other – and honour is satisfied. Meanwhile, if a person is near death, a sacrifice might be made to the ancestral spirits, so that they can welcome the about to depart person with open arms and protect them from harm. This custom of sacrifice and near-death feast is one that some African communities carry on in the UK. It is common enough for caring staff to need to know about it, understand it and help it to take place.

Customs around death

After the death, in African communities, funerals take place very quickly, usually burial. They also often lead to a period of mourning for the widow or widower, who may have to wear old clothes, sleep in different places (particularly widows, to keep them away from the spirit of their deceased husbands) and live a restricted life before coming out of mourning and often remarrying – in the case of a widow this is frequently a brother or relative of the deceased husband. This custom of marriage again within the same family is widespread in parts of Africa and is similar to the custom of levirate marriage in ancient Judaism, where a widow marries her deceased husband's brother if she is childless, so that the ensuing first child can be viewed as the child of the first husband for inheritance and name purposes. In African custom, the reasons may be much the same – certainly property brought into a family by a bride will be desirable to the deceased husband's family.

In parts of Africa, some months or years after the burial, a second ceremony takes place, making the grave firm, where the whole community attends, sings, dances and drinks beer, and prayers and sacrifices are made to ensure the dead person stays in the spirit world, with the living-dead, and does not become a troublesome or dissatisfied ghost who gives grief to the living. It is also often after that ceremony that a widower is free to remarry.

Afro-Caribbean funerals

These are usually lengthy joyous affairs with a huge attendance from the entire community. Everyone comes, food is provided for the bereaved family, children are part of the service and there are loud expressions of grief and tears at the service itself.

Some close relatives wear sashes around themselves 'to ease the pain in the stomach' caused by their loss, and they throw money into the coffin frequently to help the person on their way. The burial is conducted by the congregation, with everyone taking part, and a second ceremony often takes place nine days later to help the spirits find rest.

Although the service often seems joyous to an outsider, with uplifting gospel singing and a sense of rejoicing at the end of pain and sorrow, this should not be mistaken for a lack of true feelings of grief. The sashes are one sign, as are the lamentation and tears. The gifts of food, the presence of the wider community, the saying of words of comfort to the bereaved, and the fact that the bereaved are supported out of the church and cemetery and over a long period, are clear signs of the recognition of human grief and the need for comfort, along with joy in the going over to 'the other side'.

5

Islam

The Muslim population of the UK is growing rapidly, and some have argued that the numbers of people who attend the mosque regularly will shortly be more than those who attend church. With the rapid rise of the numbers of Muslims in the UK, and particularly with a view that is commonplace amongst many people in Britain that all Muslims are 'fundamentalist', Islamophobia has become an increasing problem. This problem is relevant for those caring for Muslims who are dying and, with an ageing population as well as a growing birth-rate, it is becoming very common. Fears of prejudice and discrimination are now widely held amongst Muslims in Britain. One thing that staff can do to good effect is reassure the patient and his family that everything will be done to provide care in accordance with the faith and customs of the particular community concerned – a mixture, therefore, of local community customs and the general practices of Islam.

History and faith

Islam is the religion of the Muslims; it means literally 'submission', signifying that a Muslim is someone who submits to God's will.

There are over 900 million Muslims in the world and Islam is growing rapidly. It is found in the Middle and Near East, large areas of Soviet Asia, Western China, Africa, Malaysia, Indonesia and throughout the Indian sub-continent. Most Muslims in Britain have their origins in the Indian sub-continent and East Africa, but there are significant groups originating from Turkey, Cyprus, Malaysia, North and Central Africa, and all over the Middle East.

Those who originate from the Indian sub-continent tend to have some similarities in custom with Hindus and Sikhs. However, the similarities are superficial, for Islam as a religion has far more in common with Judaism and Christianity than with the religions of the Indian sub-continent. It is almost militantly monotheistic. A person becoming a Muslim has to state sincerely:

> I bear witness that there is no god but God (Allah) and that Muhammad is the messenger of God.

All Muslims regard the prophet Muhammad as the final messenger of the one true God and accept the truth of the teaching of the holy Koran (Quran), taking upon themselves the code of behaviour contained in it and within the recorded sayings and deeds of Muhammad.

Most British Muslims are fairly strict about Islamic law. There is no significant liberal, non-orthodox wing of Islam in Britain, despite there being Sunni, Shi'ite, Ismaili and Ahmaddiya Muslims in the UK. The two main branches of Islam in the UK are Sunni and Shia, in a roughly 9:1 proportion to each other. The split occurred early in Islamic history. Sometimes divisions are very pronounced and hostility is felt by one for another. There are also the Ismailis (led by their hereditary imam, the Aga Khan), small in number but very influential and often the most westernised of Muslims, and the Ahmaddiya, a sect declared non-Muslim by the Pakistanis but who still claim to be Muslims themselves. There are Ahmaddiya in Britain and feeling against them from the other groups may be quite intense.

Unless a Muslim is totally 'lapsed', he is unlikely to break away from traditional Islamic attitudes to family, to modesty, to alcohol, to gambling and even to clothes. Those nursing termin-ally ill Muslims need to be very sensitive to all these attitudes, particularly to those of modesty, since nakedness and unfamiliar, western clothes can be a source of considerable distress.

The first tenet of a Muslim is that the religion of Islam was revealed by God to the prophet Muhammad in Mecca, in what is now Saudi Arabia. Muhammad was born in 570 AD but left Mecca with his followers in 622 AD to escape persecution. They went to Medina nearby and established the true meaning of Muhammad's message. Islam became a formalised, distinctive religion with its own system of government, law and rules.

The beginning of the Muslim era is the date of that journey to Medina, called the Hijra. The first year is called 1 AH, the first year after the Hijra. Muhammad died in 11 AH in Medina, but by this time Islam had spread throughout Arabia. Jerusalem, Medina and Mecca are all holy cities for Muslims (because of links either with Muhammad or Abraham), but Mecca is the most sacred of the three. Prayers are always said facing towards it, and the pilgrimage (the Hajj) is made there.

Because most Muslims in Britain have their origins in the Indian sub-continent, it is probably worth knowing that Islam first reached India early in the 8th century and that Muslim invaders established their rule in the Punjab in the 11th century, but that by the 16th century the Mughal dynasty from Central Asia had established its rule over all of North and Central India, with Delhi as their capital.

From the end of the 17th century, Mughal power diminished. Muslims were still a large part of the population, and when talk of Indian independence began in the early 20th century, some felt that they would be swamped by the Hindu majority. In 1947 the boundaries were drawn to allow a separate Muslim state of Pakistan. However, there was great violence between Hindus and Sikhs on the one side and Muslims on the other. Millions of people had to move one way or the other and hundreds of thousands were killed. The bitterness engendered was considerable and it has left an enduring legacy. A Muslim from Pakistan might find it hard to be nursed by a Hindu from India. Further complications ensued with the relationship between East and West Pakistan souring rapidly. The result was the independent state of Bangladesh, created out of the old East Pakistan. Relationships between the two are still fragile.

Muslims believe Muhammad was the last in a long line of prophets and that he completed everything that had gone before. The patriarchs of Judaism, along with Moses, David, Jesus, John the Baptist and others, are thought to be forerunners of Muhammad, but their messages were distorted by those who heard them at the time. Muhammad himself was an 'ordinary man', no mediator between human beings and God, and taught that all men and women are called to Allah's service to try to live perfectly following the Koran.

The religious duties incumbent on a practising Muslim are the five 'pillars' of Islam:

- faith in God
- daily prayer
- fasting during Ramadan
- giving alms
- making a pilgrimage to Mecca.

In Islamic thought, each person is considered to be entrusted with a certain portion of material goods to be used in God's service.

As well as the Koran, there is the Sharia, the Islamic legal system based upon the Koran and the sayings and deeds of Muhammad. The Sharia is a detailed code which covers almost every aspect of life from personal conduct to inheritance, from religious obligations to laws of property and crime. The combination of the Koran and the Sharia, with the deeds and sayings of the prophet Muhammad, provides guidance for Muslims in all possible situations. There is no division between secular and religious – all issues are subject to religious law.

Prayer and ritual purification

Every Muslim says certain prayers five times a day at set times: after dawn, at noon, mid-afternoon, just after sunset and at night. In Britain, daylight hours vary and so times for prayers (namaz or salat) are affected. The first prayer could be as early as 3 am in midsummer and the last at 11 pm, whilst in winter the prayer times run very close together.

Before prayer, Muslims wash. They stand on clean ground (or on a mat), facing Mecca (south-east in Britain). Shoes are removed and heads covered before prayer begins, and there are specified movements at different points in prayer: kneeling, touching the ground with the forehead and so on.

Hospitals and hospices may find that a compass is a useful acquisition to make sure the patient is facing east. A prayer mat might come in handy as well, as some Muslims may not bring their own.

A Muslim who is terminally ill will almost certainly wish to carry on with the ritual of daily prayers as long as possible, even though technically the seriously ill are exempt. Times will have to be ascertained and some privacy ensured. Best of all would be a small side-room into which a bed or chair can be wheeled. Failing that, curtains round the bed are a help. However, it must be borne in mind that washing has to take place before prayer. The Koran commands washing some parts of the body in running water before prayer. These are: face, ears, forehead, feet, hands and arms to the elbows. The nose is to be cleaned by sniffing up water and the mouth rinsed out.

Muslims also wash their private parts with running water after urinating or defecation, and cannot pray unless this is done. A bed-ridden Muslim may wish to be given a thorough wash with water poured from a jug after using a bed-pan. There are other circumstances when Muslims have to wash completely before prayer: both sexes after sexual intercourse, men after a nocturnal emission and women at the end of a period.

Friday is the holy day for Muslims. All males over the age of 12 go to the mosque. Except for Ismailis, Muslim women do not normally go to the mosque, but say the usual prayers at home. Some mosques provide a separate prayer room for women. It is important to know the attitudes of the particular Muslim women being nursed, as the degree of a sense of deprivation from public worship will vary considerably.

Fasting

Fasting during Ramadan is incumbent on all healthy Muslims over the age of 12. Before Ramadan begins, disputes, ill-feelings and problems have to be sorted out. Many Muslims who are terminally ill feel particularly strongly about Ramadan, as it becomes a personal, last, sorting out session. Although the seriously ill are not required to fast, Ramadan is nevertheless likely to be of considerable importance to them. Normally the rule is that the elderly and those in poor health do not fast for the whole month but should fast a little if they can. Some terminally ill Muslim patients may elect to do that. Alternatively they may wish to make charitable gifts to make up for fast-days they have missed. If Muslim patients are fasting even for a few days, special arrangements will need to be made for them. They will need a meal before dawn and another after sunset, as well as a glass of water and a bowl to rinse out their mouths before prayer.

It is worth mentioning that, even when very ill, devout Muslims may insist on fasting for part of Ramadan at least. This would include not taking anything into their bodies by mouth, nose, injection or suppository, from dawn to sunset. It can make pain control almost impossible and is a source of considerable headache to carers. Nevertheless, it obviously gives comfort to the patient, who must be left to make up his own mind without undue pressure from healthcare staff. Often the local imam can be helpful here. Although imams do not always take on the pastoral role of the Christian clergy, many have assumed at least part of this role, and in situations such as these will willingly come and talk to the patient and discuss whether fasting will be spiritually beneficial.

Modesty

Modesty is crucial to Muslims, who are deeply shocked by nakedness. Women are traditionally clothed from head to foot except for their faces, and clothes conceal the shape of their bodies. Muslim women are also fully dressed at night (in clothes similar to their daytime ones, but loosened) and will expect to be able to remain fully clothed within a hospital or a hospice.

Men are also extremely modest. They are obliged to be covered from waist to knee and nudity, even in the presence of other men, is seen as offensive. Muslim men cover their heads for prayer and for ceremonies such as marriages and funerals. However, older and devout men may wish to keep their heads covered at all times, a desire which should be respected by those caring for them.

The strong desire for modesty may cause considerable problems in a hospital or hospice setting. Women often react strongly to male doctors or nurses and find the contact humiliating, rendering them unclean. Muslim women should always be examined and treated by women doctors and nurses and men by men. Sensitivity in this area can avoid a great many problems. There can be a funny side to it, however; older Muslim men are often very dubious about female nurses and female doctors in positions of authority – they are thought of as having physical contact with 'strange men' and must therefore be of very low status. I was highly amused, a few years ago, to hear a very grand woman doctor recently described as a prostitute by an elderly Muslim patient – my explanations only helped a little. It may well be easiest simply to avoid the problem, and providing female staff for Muslim women is undoubtedly essential.

Diet

Almost all Muslims observe the dietary rules. In a hospital or hospice, most will therefore follow a vegetarian diet unless halal meat can be provided. Nowadays, most healthcare institutions in the UK are well able to cope with a suitable diet, including halal meat.

Muslims eat no pork or pig products. All other meat is allowed if it is halal, killed according to Islamic law. Muslims can eat kosher meat if no halal meat is available. If kosher meat is given, this may need to be explained. Fish is permitted however it is killed, but any fish which has no fins and scales, except prawns, is forbidden.

Dairy products are acceptable providing that no non-halal animal rennet has been used. Alcohol is expressly forbidden and even when it is used in some drugs, such as 'cocktails', many

Muslims will object. It is always worth checking with the individual patient and family about this.

Methods of cooking and serving are also extremely important for Muslims. They cannot eat food that has touched forbidden food. Utensils that have been used for ham, say, and then salad without washing in between render the salad forbidden. Like orthodox Jews and strict Hindus and Sikhs, some Muslims will refuse all food that has not been cooked and served separately. Nursing staff must be aware of this and be prepared to get special food in. Any doubts in this area need to be discussed with the patient and his family.

Muslim festivals

Apart from Friday and Ramadan, which are well known, Islam has other festivals. They occur, as Ramadan does, at different times each year because the Islamic calendar is a lunar one; this means 354 days each year instead of 365, so festivals slip back 11 days each year.

The two most important festivals for our purposes are Id-ul-Fitr, which marks the end of Ramadan, and Id-ul-Azha, which commemorates the Hajj and Abraham's willingness to sacrifice his son (Ishmael, not Isaac, in Islamic tradition). Both these 'Ids' are of great importance, comparable with Christmas and Easter in Christianity. They are celebrated with prayer, visits to family, exchanging gifts, sending of cards and the giving of alms.

When Muslims are terminally ill in a hospital or hospice during Id, much can be done to help. If it is at all possible to go home, that would usually be hugely appreciated. If that is impossible for whatever reason, then – if practicable – routine tests and examinations should be avoided on Id and the family should be encouraged to come in, bearing gifts, cards and special food. Other patients, staff and families should be encouraged to wish the Muslim patient and his family a happy Id.

Attitudes to life and death

Like Christians and many Jews, Muslims believe in life after death merely as one stage in God's plan for humanity. So the death of a beloved person is seen as a temporary separation and, since the death is God's will, struggle and recrimination are wrong. Devout and pious Muslims believe that death is part of God's plan and that one's duty is to try to accept whatever God sends, surrendering to His will, however difficult. It is for this reason that some very pious Muslims discipline themselves to show no emotion at a death, because open crying would suggest rebellion against God's will. It is, however, much more common to find grief being displayed openly, crying and weeping being the order of the day. All friends and relatives are duty bound to visit the bereaved and to comfort them.

Muslims also believe in bodily resurrection at the time of the coming of the Messiah (who has not come yet, Jesus being thought of as one of the great teachers of the six eras of the law givers – Adam, Noah, Abraham, Moses, Jesus and Muhammad). The present era is that of Muhammad and Islam, but the future – and seventh – era is that of the time of the Messiah when no law will be necessary because truth will prevail everywhere. At that time there will be physical resurrection for all people (or Muslims), although the Ismailis do not believe in that. They believe in purely spiritual resurrection, the life of the spirit in the hereafter. For Ismailis, resurrection is an intellectual concept – only the mind survives and knowledge is the reward of Heaven.

When a Muslim dies

A religious leader – an imam or maulana – is not necessary when a Muslim is dying: family members often stay by the bed and pray. They usually perform all the rites and ceremonies as well, saying, first of all, as a statement of faith in all circumstances:

There is no god but Allah, and Muhammad is His prophet.

These are the last words a Muslim should say. If possible, the dying Muslim should sit or lie with his face turned towards Mecca, whilst another Muslim whispers the call to prayer into his ear. Family members recite prayers, but there is no confession. If there is no family around, any practising Muslim can help. The best thing, if there is no Muslim chaplain on call, is to contact the nearest mosque and ask for someone to come.

Once a Muslim has died, it is as well to be aware that many Muslims are fussy about who touches the body (rather like Jews). Ideally, it should not be touched by non-Muslims but, if it is essential, non-Muslims should wear disposable gloves to prevent actual contact. If the family is willing, the eyes should be closed, limbs straightened and the head turned towards the right shoulder (in order to bury the body with the face turned to Mecca). The body should be wrapped in a plain sheet, unwashed.

In normal circumstances, where Muslims are carrying out the procedures for themselves, the body is straightened, the eyes closed, the feet tied together with a thread around the toes and the face bandaged so as to keep the mouth closed. The body is then taken home or to the mosque and washed, usually by the family. Women wash a female, men a male corpse. Camphor is often put in the armpits and in the orifices. The body is clothed in clean white cotton garments: a seamless shirt, wrapping and a covering sheet. The arms are placed across the chest. Those who have been on the Hajj to Mecca may have brought back a white cotton shroud.

Muslims are buried, never cremated. The funeral takes place as soon as possible, usually within 24 hours. After the body is washed, passages from the Koran are read and the family prays. The body is then taken to the mosque or graveside for prayers before the actual burial. Muslims would not usually be buried in a coffin, but in Britain it is a requirement as is the marking of a grave (in Islamic law, the grave is unmarked). Some local authorities provide a special area for Muslims, but where this provision is not made its lack can cause considerable distress to the family who may need a lot of support in dealing with the undertakers.

After the funeral

Mourning usually lasts for around a month, and relatives and friends visit and provide comfort and support. They talk about the person who has died, extolling his or her virtues and sharing the loss. Usually the family stays at home for the first three days after the funeral. They do not cook, but are brought food by friends and relatives.

For 40 days the grave is visited on Fridays and alms distributed to the poor. A widow should modify her behaviour for 130 days, staying indoors unless absolutely necessary and wearing plain clothes and no jewellery.

Muslim patients do not usually have great problems in facing death. However, rituals are important and great comfort and support are gained from carrying out as much religious practice as possible. This is particularly important in a social climate where Muslims feel that the majority is somehow stacked up against them – the more that can be done to offer support and understanding, plus basic knowledge, the more relaxed a Muslim patient and his family will be.

6

Hinduism

History and faith

Hinduism is more than a religion. Some argue that it is a series of '...isms', a collection of different, very early religions somehow taken over and incorporated into one. Others say that it is a way of life and that that way of life has itself varied from place to place. It is practised fairly widely in Britain. There are active Hindu societies in many of our big cities, and there are Hindu temples and cultural groups.

Hinduism is a very ancient religion; no-one is certain of its exact age. It has thousands of gods and goddesses, but most Hindus would argue that these are all manifestations of one God in many different forms. Indeed, Hindu scholars will often argue that most religions have different manifestations of their God (they often cite Christianity with its Father, Son and Holy Ghost) and that the accusation that Hinduism is not monotheistic, whilst other religions are, is plainly absurd. This is a problem that nursing staff sometimes have to deal with. There is, quite understandably, some resentment amongst Hindus in Britain that their religion is not taken sufficiently seriously by people of other faiths, and it is important to understand something of the Hindu pantheon.

The three supreme gods of Hinduism are Brahma the creator, Vishnu the preserver, and Shiva the destroyer and regenerator of life. However, with these go innumerable other gods. Anyone who has ever been to India will have seen the figures, statuettes and pictures of local or particularly helpful gods: Ganesh, the elephant god, frequently on the front of lorries; Kali, Shiva's wife, at the back of shops in the bazaar.

Hindus divide up into different sects whose beliefs and philosophies are quite different. The majority of Hindus in Britain are Vishnavites, that is to say that they worship principally Vishnu the preserver and his incarnations as Rama and Krishna. As Rama, Vishnu was a good king, combining beauty, bravery and justice. As Krishna, he was a charming young man who brought with him happiness and fun as well as power and justice. Some Vishnavites believe that he will come again in a future incarnation as Kaliki, when he will bring about the end of the world and destroy evil forever. Most Hindu religious literature dates from three or four millennia ago at the earliest – there are the Vedas, the Upanishads, the Brahmanas and the long epics of the Bhagavad Gita based on the Nahabharata and the Ramayana.

There is no standard way for Hindus to worship. Some meditate quietly, while others go to the temple once or twice a week or even once or twice a day. Some combine their meditation, prayer and physical exercise into a particular discipline, called Hatha Yoga. Yoga itself, as a method of relaxation at least, is very well known in Britain. However, there is a basic philosophy which is more or less shared, if not expressed, by most Hindus. The Hindu design for living suggests that man's life should be divided into four parts.

1 Brahmacharya, the period of education.
2 Garhasthya, the period of working in the world.
3 Vanapastha, the retreat, ready for the loosening of ties and worldly attachments.
4 Pravrajya or yati, the awaiting of freedom through death.

For the purposes of this book, stages three and four are perhaps of most interest. In the third stage, the individual, though beginning to be aloof from this world, still keeps in touch with it by imparting to it his worldly wisdom. In the fourth stage, those relationships are gradually severed so that the spirit can be released to unite with the Supreme Being. The individual is not supposed to allow things to come to a sudden halt, but is to reach the stage of renunciation gracefully. For our purposes, if that stage has been carried out to good effect, bringing comfort to dying Hindus becomes very much easier. The stages of life suggest that there is a time for all things, and the Hindu believes in a return to earth in either a better or worse form according to one's karma.

The doctrine of karma is often wrongly explained in the West. It is not pure fatalism, but it represents the idea that what the individual does in this world affects what will happen to him in the next. Similarly, his position or life in this world is at least partly the result of actions in the life before. More disturbing to some of us, health was often considered to be the reward for living by religious and moral laws.

There is a defined science of life which affects Hindu medicine very considerably. This is Ayurveda, a well-defined philosophy shared by physicians and patients. A routine is advocated, with regular diet, sleep, defecation, cleanliness of body and clothing, and moderation in physical exercise and sexual indulgence – these form a large part of the beliefs of Hindu medicine. A Hindu patient may well adhere to much of this and want to discuss aspects of care. In some cases he may be worried by the thought that this final illness is, in some way, his fault and may indeed feel a sense of guilt.

Most Hindus living in Britain have been considerably influenced by our western theories about what causes illness and infection, though equally there has been considerable influence from Ayurvedic medicine within holistic approaches to health-care – now very widely accepted. Nurses may well find themselves in great philosophical difficulties when dealing with worried Hindu patients, since attitudes to health and sickness can be so very different. It is always as well to call in a Hindu priest or local members of the Hindu society, if this is causing concern. Most Hindus will, however, regard their death as insignificant because of their certainty of being at one with God in their life after death.

One other facet of Hindu belief that must be mentioned is the caste system. Although it is now illegal in modern India to discriminate on the basis of caste, the system still has a very strong hold, and people's lives are far more affected by it than many of them would care to admit. The importance given to caste varies from community to community, but in all of them the Brahmins (the priests) are top of the pile, and the Harijans (the untouchables) at the bottom. Menstruating women and mourners are also temporarily untouchable because of their ritual impurity.

Ritual purification

Hindus believe that purification of the body is as necessary as purification of the mind. They try to bathe in running water daily. Bathing in a bath of water, as we often do, strikes them as disgusting since the water from which one emerges is not clean. Running water, such as a stream or a shower, is what is considered best, and preferably showering should happen first thing in the morning. This is particularly true for older Hindus, who like to bathe early in the day before saying their prayers, even if they are very ill, and may need a lot of help to achieve it. Hindu belief suggests that bathing does not only render one physically clean but also spiritually clean, so a dying patient might be especially eager to carry out this religious duty. It is also quite often the case that a patient going for surgery will be particularly keen to shower early on in the day, as bathing is to be undertaken on auspicious occasions as well as in the normal run of things.

Food restrictions, fasting and modesty

Washing is an important part of Hindu life. Washing hands and rinsing the mouth before and after meals are considered essential, and strict cleanliness in the handling and preparation of food is always observed. Many Hindus ask for food from home for both hygiene and taboo reasons. Although a hospital can usually cope with the total ban on beef and indeed with the large number of Hindus (especially women) who are vegetarian, there are not so many which could handle the taboo on beef which stretches to not eating food touched by it in cooking or serving. Equally, few hospitals could guarantee production of food by Hindus of the same caste as the patient. It is crucial that all these facets of dietary restriction are borne in mind, as it is all too easy otherwise to reassure patients of the fitness of food which, by their standard, is far from being acceptable.

Fasting is not uncommon amongst Hindu women, especially widows and elderly women. For special festivals, men and women fast on regular days of the week. In the case of patients who are dying, the effects of long fasting on fluid balances and pain relieving drugs need to be explained. It may be that the family will discourage the patient from fasting. On the other hand, if fasting has been their normal practice, it may be as well to let it continue where possible since it is a genuine expression of religious feeling. Conflict between nurses and patient should be avoided; ultimately the decision on whether or not to fast must be the patient's.

There may be problems with modesty rules as well. Hindu women, in particular, are often reluctant to undress for examination. Total privacy for bed baths, for instance, is essential. Many Hindu women would be shocked at being given a bath by a male nurse, and many Hindu men by a female nurse. This is something which must be respected. Disregard for modesty can cause extreme distress and is simply not justifiable. Sensitivity to it can help to elicit information which is often otherwise quite hard to obtain.

Discomfort, pain and problems in the genito-urinary and bowel areas are usually not spoken about by Hindus, and in terminal illness with painkilling drugs and their attendant constipation problems, this can be a cause of considerable concern. These areas are particularly not mentioned if the spouse is present; yet the Carak Samhita, the guide to healthcare for Hindus, says that a physician may not attend a woman in the absence of her husband or guardian. Quite apart from this, strong families visit constantly and the patient will want his family around. Conversations about intimate details of pain and constipation are therefore often extremely difficult.

Hindu worship

Most Hindus need time for meditation and prayer and this requirement will undoubtedly continue in terminal illness. The elderly often use the early morning, while younger people tend to have no fixed time. What may often be required, however, is somewhere to go to be alone. Even if the bed has to be wheeled into another room, the need to be alone for meditation is considerable amongst some Hindus. Others will find it quite acceptable to pray in bed. In either case, small images or pictures of gods may be kept under the pillow or by the bed, as may praying beads and blessings (flowers, charms) and amulets. Since the Hindu pantheon is a large one, there may be any number of small figurines, for some Hindus adopt one favourite god while others choose to worship several. All this is difficult for many westerners and can only be understood in terms of all the gods being expressions, in one form or another, of one God. However difficult western Europeans find the theology of Hinduism, they must respect the enormous comfort that Hindus derive from their gods and they must recognise Hinduism as a religion, and a philosophy, which brings support and help to its adherents. It is still all too common to hear Christian nurses trying to convince those with eastern faiths that their religions are in some way inferior and of less value. No-one who knew anything serious about Hinduism, with its complex and highly developed philosophy of life, could consider it inferior; they might, however, legitimately find it confusing.

Last offices

Hindu priests (priests are called pandits), Brahmins, can be very helpful. They will often come in to help dying patients with their acts of worship, called puja. They will also help the dying patient to accept death philosophically, an acceptance which is a strong feature of Hindu attitudes. The whole Hindu religious outlook is geared to the acceptance of the inevitable (and sometimes, sadly, of the avoidable as well). Families and friends will weep, but the death is accepted without the manifestations of obvious anger which characterise Judaism, Christianity and Islam.

Customs in death vary. Some place the body on the floor and light lamps while incense burns. Others do neither of these. However, in all cases cremation is the order of the day whether on the burning ghats of the Ganges or in the suburban crematoria of England. Even there, Ganges water will usually be present.

After a death, there is a ceremony called Sreda, when food offerings are brought to the Brahmins who perform some rites for the dead. There is usually a time of isolation or segregation at this time, and the chief mourners go into a form of seclusion or retirement. Nevertheless, grief is expressed openly with physical gestures; hands are held and people embrace, for such physical comfort is considered very important to those who survive.

Usually there is no restriction on non-Hindus handling the body, provided it is wrapped in a plain sheet. However, post-mortems are often considered extremely objectionable and deeply disrespectful to the dead. It is often difficult to persuade Hindu families of the need for a post-mortem and it is an issue which needs to be handled with great sensitivity because the act of opening up the body is considered to be disrespectful to the dead person and his family.

In conclusion, Hindu beliefs and practices vary considerably and this can only be the roughest of outlines. At the same time, it is important to recognise a totally different attitude to human life and to treat it with respect. This in itself will increase the patient's confidence in the nurse. In most cases, where at all possible, it is advisable to ask the patient or the family the nature of the particular religious observances to be carried out.

7

Sikhism

History and faith

The Sikh community in Britain has been growing and, like many
other relatively recent immigrant groups, is now ageing. It is
therefore going to be more and more necessary for nursing staff
to know what to do when a Sikh patient dies. A very basic
understanding of what Sikhism is has become essential, nor is it
necessarily all that easy. There is great controversy amongst
academic historians of religion who say that Sikhism is either an
offshoot of Hinduism or that it is Hinduism heavily influenced
by Islam. In fact, neither is wholly true. It is, in a sense, an
offshoot of Hinduism in that it grew up amongst people who
had previously been Hindus, but they became strongly disaffected from it, regarding some parts of it as positively dangerous
and other elements as unnecessarily ritualistic.

The Sikh religion is monotheistic and was founded by Guru
Nanak (1469–1533). Sikh means disciple or follower, and it is as
followers of Guru Nanak and his nine successors that the Sikhs
became an independent religious body. Guru Nanak had been
born a Hindu and was shocked by many of the features of
contemporary Hinduism. He particularly deplored the caste
system and the power and influence of the priesthood. His aim

was to return to the essentials of religion, to the relationship of each individual with his God, to the search for a virtuous life and to the idea that only by doing good in this life was there a route to salvation. Much of this is highly individual and personal, there being a strong element of personal religion within Sikhism as each individual strives to know God. There is a strong community aspect to Sikhism as well and the life of the community in the gurdwara (Sikh temple), where all Sikhs gather, is seen as one of group activity, especially eating together.

Sikhism has no priesthood at all and the communities run their own gurdwaras, providing services for all those who need them. In Britain, the gurdwara has become even more important than it was in India because it is, amongst other things, a clearing house for information as well as the place where the whole community can meet to celebrate births, engagements, marriages, birthdays and so on. The gurdwara is also a place of hospitality for travellers and visitors; anyone may stay the night there and eat there free of charge. This applies both to Sikhs and non-Sikhs and illustrates just how strong the tradition of hospitality is in Sikhism. Several gurdwaras in Britain now serve daily meals for unemployed or homeless people, wholly in accordance with the teachings of Guru Nanak and his successors. Action is to be taken in this world with no thought for the next. Indeed, Guru Nanak and his successors stressed involvement in this world, families, friends and community, and service to the community instead of asceticism, self-imposed suffering, deprivation and celibacy as one might find in some schools of Hindu thought.

Guru Nanak was followed by nine gurus who consolidated his original work. The last was Guru Gobind Singh (1675–1708) who tried to form the Sikhs into a recognisable people or group. He wanted to strengthen them as a military fellowship (probably because they were then, and had been for some time, fighting off the Mughal invaders) and he therefore gave them five symbols which initiated men and women were to wear. The equality of the sexes was something which Guru Nanak had started but which Guru Gobind Singh did much to consolidate.

The five K symbols

The symbols of faith include the Kesh, the Kangha, the Kara, the Kirpan and the Kaccha.

Kesh: Uncut hair

This is usually left long and in a bun by both men and women, but men cover it with a turban while women tend merely to wear it up, with the exception of a few elderly and very pious Sikh women who wear black turbans.

Kangha: A comb

The bun (jura) is kept in place with a small wooden or plastic semi-circular comb, the kangha, which is of major significance to the Sikhs. They will want to have it with them always and if for some reason it cannot be in their hair, as in the case of someone who has had an operation on the head or has had chemotherapy leading to severe hair loss, then the kangha should be close by and should never be taken away by hospital staff without express instruction.

Kara: The steel bangle

Even the most assimilated Sikhs, such as those who have cut their hair, wear a steel bangle on their right wrist. Left-handed people wear the bangle on the left wrist. In origin the kara was supposed to protect the military Sikh from the bowstring cutting into him, but now it is supposed to represent the unity of God by virtue of its circular shape. An adult initiated Sikh never removes his kara, and it is a source of considerable distress even to non-observant Sikhs if the kara is removed for an operation or for any other reason. Before any surgery, the kara should be covered with tape, as a wedding ring is, and not be removed. In the very rare cases where removal is essential, such as for surgery on that part of the arm, the reasons should be carefully explained and the patient encouraged to wear it on the other wrist or keep it under the pillow or in a pocket.

Kirpan: The symbolic dagger

This is the dagger to symbolise the Sikh's readiness to fight in self-defence and to protect the poor and oppressed. It varies considerably in appearance, from a tiny symbolic dagger to a long sword, and it is worn under the clothes in a cloth sheath (gatra) over the right shoulder and under the left arm at waist level. As with the kara, left-handed people wear the kirpan the other way round. In Britain, most Sikhs wear a very small kirpan or a brooch or pendant with a kirpan shape and some even have a kirpan engraved on the side of their kangha, but that is not universal and there are some men and women who wear a six-inch or more long kirpan in the gurdwara on special occasions.

It is important to realise that those who do wear the kirpan wear it all the time, in bed, in the shower and everywhere. Sadly, it has been all too common for nursing staff to try and remove the kirpan from Sikh patients at night on the grounds that it is dangerous. This causes immense and unnecessary distress and often discourages Sikh patients from seeking help when they need it. Particularly in the case of dying patients, no such restrictions should be applied by the staff. If for any really good reason the kirpan does have to be removed, then it must be kept within the sight of the patient and the issue discussed with the patient and his family.

Kaccha: Special underpants or shorts

These were probably invented to replace the traditional dhoti (a length of cloth wound round the legs) to make for easier movement in battle. However, they have come to be regarded by Sikhs as a symbol of modesty and sexual morality. Although many Sikhs would now wear ordinary underpants instead of the traditional knee-length kaccha as invented by Guru Gobind Singh, nevertheless they would be thought to have the same significance and the Sikh patient might well resist having to remove them completely. For instance, in the Punjab, Sikh women often give birth to children with one leg in one hole of the kaccha, and Sikhs usually wear a pair of kaccha at night and in the shower, changing the wet ones for clean, dry ones after-wards. A fairly modest Sikh would be careful never to remove the kaccha completely when changing them, but would have one leg in the new pair before removing the old ones entirely. This is extremely important in hospitals where ill Sikhs are concerned. This worry about modesty is even more common amongst older Sikhs, and with a dying patient it is crucial to respect this concern and to help to keep a leg in the kaccha, even when using a bedpan or having a bed bath.

Scripture

The holy book of the Sikhs is called the Guru Granth Sahib. Granth means anthology, and before he died, Guru Gobind Singh gave the Guru Granth Sahib to the Sikhs as their new guru, since there would be no more human gurus. The Guru Granth Sahib became the focal point of the gurdwara and formed the basis for all Sikh ceremonies. It is treated with love and reverence and passages from it are learned by heart, which dying patients in hospital might well want to hear if someone from the local gurdwara can be contacted to help. It is written in Punjabi in the Sikh special alphabet, Gurmukhi, which all Sikhs learn in order to be able to read and under-stand their Guru Granth Sahib. These lessons take place in the gurdwara, as do most of the other Sikh ceremonies, and the dying Sikh patient is likely to feel very cut off from his own community by virtue of not being able to get to the gurdwara. In most instances the local gurdwara (the granthi, or reader, is the person in charge there in many cases) will send people round to sit with the dying person if there is no available family.

However, there is also a tradition of private prayer which many devout Sikhs follow. They get up very early and shower (there is a general eastern preference for washing in running water rather than in a bath) and then pray for one or two hours before breakfast. Although the early start may be difficult to organise and is probably unnecessary, it would often be greatly appreciated by a Sikh patient who cannot easily get out of bed and is very ill, if the offer was made to help him wash before praying. Privacy whilst actually praying is also much appreciated. If nothing better can be arranged, then curtains pulled around the bed will suffice, but a side ward would be even better and many Sikh and Hindu patients clearly appreciate that particular need for privacy being met.

Food restrictions

There are some food restrictions which are binding upon Sikhs. The only one which is universal is the prohibition against eating meat that is halal (killed in the approved way for Muslims). The relationship between Muslims and Sikhs was not always an easy one. However, many Sikhs, particularly women, follow the Hindu tradition of vegetarianism, including not eating eggs which are regarded as a source of life. Amongst non-vegetarian Sikhs, very few eat beef, again following a Hindu tradition, and quite a few will not eat pork. Sikhs originating from East Africa tend to be less concerned about food restrictions than Sikhs from the Indian sub-continent. There is some evidence that, with the increasing political militancy of some Sikhs in the Punjab, the tradition is veering more towards vegetarianism. Alcohol is forbidden to Sikhs and the new drinking habits amongst some of the younger Sikh men in Britain are deeply frowned on by older, more conservative community leaders. This ban can cause some problems with dying patients. Some hospitals and hospices offer a drink of beer or spirits to their dying (and other) patients. In many cases, this would be deeply offensive to Sikhs and should be avoided. Tobacco is also expressly forbidden by Guru Gobind Singh and is found disgusting by many Sikhs.

Death and the afterlife

Sikh and Hindu beliefs are very similar about the doctrine of reincarnation which affects attitudes to death quite substantially. Each soul goes through many cycles of birth and rebirth. Death is not, therefore, a frightening thing, but the ultimate aim is for each soul to reach perfection and so to be reunited with God and to be able to avoid having to come back into this world. This is slightly at odds with the strong ideal of communal service held by Sikhism and the devotion to the actions of this life. Nevertheless, Sikhs believe in the doctrine of karma, as Hindus do, with its cycle of reward and punishment for all thoughts and deeds. Each person's life in this world is determined by their behaviour in their last life and what they do now influences the next life, and so on. Unlike Hinduism, Sikhs believe that the cycle can be altered by good actions in life and that God's grace can be extended to human beings beyond what they might have expected. This is a difficult doctrine for those brought up in western religions to grasp. It has taken from Islam a strong sense of the individual's responsibility for his own actions, but at the same time has inherited the doctrine of karma from Hinduism and believes that each life one lives in this world influences the next.

Because of the doctrine of reincarnation, Sikhs tend not to be very scared of death, unless they feel that their next life is likely to be particularly dreadful. This often makes their actual death much easier, and comfort can often be given by arranging to have readings from the Guru Granth Sahib and by encouraging private prayer.

Last offices

Where possible, the dying Sikh's family will remain and tell the nursing staff what is required. In all Asian traditions, the family is responsible for all the last offices and they may wish to continue this in Britain. If that is the case, all that the nurses should do, in consultation with the family, is to close the eyes, straighten out the limbs and wrap the body in a plain sheet without any religious emblem on it. The normal Sikh practice is for the family to wash and dress the body. Each Sikh is cremated wearing the five K symbols listed above. Men are wrapped in a white cotton shroud with a turban and women are wrapped in red if young and white if older. Bodies of still-born children should be given to the parents for funeral rites to be carried out. In these cases, it is usually a burial rather than a cremation.

Cremation should take place as soon as possible and usually occurs within 24 hours of death in India. Families often appreciate some help in convincing the undertaker that there is a great degree of urgency in this matter. There are various ways in which the funeral takes place in Britain, but the most common is for the coffin to go first to the family home and to be opened for people to pay their last respects. It then either goes to the gurdwara for the bulk of the service or to the crematorium direct where the service is to be held. One of the most important duties of the heir to the dead person (usually, but not always, the eldest son) is to light the funeral pyre. The nearest that can be achieved in Britain is the pushing of the button at the crematorium for the curtains to close or for the coffin to move towards the doors of the furnace. The ashes are collected and scattered in a river or in the sea, although they are quite often taken by a family member to the Punjab and scattered there, often at the River Sutlej at Anandpur where Sikhism was founded by Guru Nanak.

After the cremation the family, plus friends, go back to the gurdwara for more prayers, although these are usually fairly brief, before going home. While they may wash at the gurdwara, it is also likely that they will have a shower when they get home.

On the first day after the death, friends provide the family with food, and in the 10 to 13 days following the death, the whole family remains in mourning. Relatives and friends come and visit to bring comfort and support. The home may have one room turned temporarily into a temple – where an akhand path, a complete reading of the Guru Granth Sahib, takes place. It can be done at the gurdwara, but if it is at home then a room is cleared of all furniture and everything is replaced with a covered dais (manji) with a canopy on top (palki). There are cushions on the dais and the Guru Granth Sahib is set on the cushions. People coming into the room remove their shoes and have their heads covered with a turban, veil or piece of clean cloth. They kneel before the Guru Granth Sahib, put some money at the bottom of the dais as a contribution towards the communal food and for the poor and then sit on the floor to hear the scripture being read, usually by elders. Family members will certainly try to be present for at least part of the reading.

Sometimes members of the family, particularly women, will not eat until after the cremation has taken place. Women wear white as a sign of mourning. (White appears to have been an almost universal colour of mourning until the mediaeval period in Europe, when black came in.)

After 10 to 13 days, a special ceremony called Bhog is held to mark the end of official mourning. A complete reading of the Guru Granth Sahib takes place either at home or at the gurdwara. A distribution of karah parshad, Sikh holy food, a combination of flour, honey and milk, is made. If the dead person was the head of the family, a turban is placed on the eldest son's head to show he is now head of the family. Then everyone has a communal meal (langar) before life goes back to normal, although the adjustment can take a considerable time. If all this takes place at home, the home temple is dismantled after the Bhog ceremony and the room goes back to normal, though a lamp may be kept lit for some weeks in memory of the person who has died.

8

Buddhism

History and faith

Buddhism is the major religion in Burma, Bhutan, Nepal, Sikkim, Sri Lanka, Thailand and Tibet. It is also found increasingly in India, parts of Africa and Japan, and in the West. There are growing numbers of Buddhists in Britain, from a variety of different schools, and it is likely that they will become one of the larger religious minorities in the near future.

Buddhism was founded on the Indian sub-continent about 2500 years ago by Siddhartha Gautama (an Indian prince), probably in what is now Nepal. He was born in about 560 BC and became deeply troubled by the miseries of life amongst the ordinary people around him in India. He decided to try to help his people find happiness and contentment by searching for truth. The answer – or perhaps more accurately the beginning of the answer – was the four noble truths which Gautama discovered as he sat on a river bank under a sacred fig tree. From that point on he was called Buddha which means the enlightened or awakened one.

Buddhism is a unique religion in that it acknowledges no god as creator. It does, however, acknowledge many gods, though these are all seen as lesser beings than the Buddha himself. Some scholars would argue that it is more a way of living than a religion because of its lack of belief in a godhead. Yet it is clearly a religious discipline with a compelling philosophy. Its teaching is based on non-violence and brotherhood with a duty incumbent on its adherents to seek spiritual growth. Buddhists believe in a doctrine of rebirth – often thought, mistakenly, by westerners to be the same as reincarnation. In the Buddhist rebirth, everything changes when an individual who has lived many lives before carries on into a future life after death. Whatever someone does in this particular present life influences the next stage in the rebirth process. If the individual pays attention to the teachings of Buddhism and tries to live by them, then in each life he learns from past experiences and gradually progresses towards perfection, Nirvana. The achievement of Nirvana implies the attainment of the infinite state of perfection where there is no selfishness and no awareness of one's own separate identity. At the same time, there should be no repression of one's true need for personal spiritual growth.

It is a discipline of extreme rigour, beginning by requiring the following of what is known as the eightfold path, which stems from Buddha's four truths. The first noble truth is that suffering and human existence are strongly linked. The second is that suffering itself is caused by the human craving for pleasure – a craving which makes knowledge and insight difficult. The third truth is that human beings will become free of sorrow by destroying 'unskilful states of mind' – those which result in unpleasant consequences. The fourth teaches the noble eight-fold path: that right understanding, aspiration, speech, action, livelihood, effort, thought and meditation will lead to the end of the state of suffering. Buddha describes this ideal state of perfect freedom and peace without suffering as Nirvana. It is not like Heaven, however, a place which is 'other'. It is, instead, more like a state or quality of mind. Nevertheless, the Buddhist concept of Nirvana has had its influence on liberal Christian and Jewish concepts of Heaven. Rather than being away, distant and beyond, Nirvana lies within the individual and is achievable by each person in his or her own way.

The eightfold path of Buddhism is a lifelong way of living, approaching and perceiving the world.

1 The Buddhist tries to acquire a complete understanding of life.
2 The Buddhist aims to develop the right outlook and the right motives.
3 The Buddhist tries to practise right speech which implies no lying, slandering, gossip or harsh speech.
4 The Buddhist aims to carry out perfect conduct. This involves being and doing good as well as ceasing to be and to perform evil. A Buddhist must be careful not to take life. A Buddhist must refrain from extremes. A Buddhist must not be dishonest or deceitful.
5 A Buddhist tries to earn his or her living in a manner appropriate to Buddhist teaching. This is called right livelihood.
6 A Buddhist tries to practise right effort which means developing self-discipline.
7 A Buddhist tries to develop right-mindedness by meditation which develops his or her awareness of self and others and also encourages positive emotions of warmth, love and peace.
8 A Buddhist aims to practise perfect meditation, which leads to complete enlightenment. This meditation is a one-pointedness of mind which is focused in the present moment. It is often described as direct knowing. Buddhist techniques of concentration and meditation have something in common with the yoga of Hinduism, and there are various other disciplines used.

Different forms of Buddhism

There are two major schools of Buddhism, geographically divided but generally co-existing peacefully.

The southern school, Theravada or the Teaching of the Elders, is found in Burma, Laos, Cambodia, Sri Lanka, Thailand and parts of India. Theravada is the only surviving branch of Hinayana, or Lesser Way, Buddhism and claims to adhere strictly to the original teaching of the Buddha, as found in the earliest texts. Some of its critics argue that it is more rigid and less rich than other Buddhist teaching.

The other main school of thought in Buddhism is the Mahayana, or Greater Way. Many Buddhists are critical of the

Mahayana school because they argue that it has adopted many unorthodox practices and is not what Buddhism should be.

Clearly the differences between the two schools are attitudinal rather than about real orthodoxies. A greater difference still exists between the two schools on the one hand and Zen Buddhism on the other. Yet Zen Buddhism is itself a branch of Mahayana Buddhism, which originated in China in the 6th century AD. It traces its roots to a teacher from India called Bodhidharma who arrived in China in 520 AD. The word Zen is a Japanese translation of a Chinese word, Chan, which is itself derived from the Indian language of Sanskrit. The Sanskrit word for Chan is Dhyana which means meditation. Zen Buddhism has influenced the Japanese martial arts such as archery, judo and samurai warrior skills, which may at first seem to be out of keeping with the peaceful nature of other Buddhist schools. On the other hand, it embraces the art of flower-arranging as well, and the Japanese tea ceremony, again unknown to other schools. There is a seriously intellectual side to Zen Buddhism, a rigorous intellectual discipline which has found many adherents in the West.

Zen Buddhism is divided into two sects: the Rinzai and Soto Zen sects. Rinzai Zen Buddhism was founded by Eisai, a 12th century teacher who went to China and developed Rinzai thinking there before establishing it in Japan on his return. Rinzai stresses the study of sutras whilst developing new techniques of meditation. Soto Zen was introduced by a follower of Eisai, Dogen, and emphasises sitting meditation in particular.

Another form of Buddhism which has a very strong following amongst westerners is Tibetan Buddhism, or Vajrayana Buddhism. This is a devotional form of Buddhism which places great emphasis on the actual moment of death. In this school, there may be a wish to hear part of the Tibetan Book of the Dead read by a Tibetan monk as death approaches.

Buddhists in the UK belong to a variety of Buddhist groups. Patients, and their families, will need to be asked about which school of Buddhism they belong to, and what their particular approach might mean for their time in a hospital or hospice setting.

Festivals, dietary rules and meditation

Festivals observed by Buddhists vary quite a lot, although Theravada Buddhism will tend particularly to stress Buddha Day in the spring. Dietary rules, disciplines and customs also vary enormously. The individual concerned will usually explain what is required, but the only certainty when caring for a Buddhist who is dying is that he will require as much time and space for meditation as possible. This can be a considerable demand, although individual Buddhists vary in how much meditation time they would like. Some Buddhists, however, are not able to meditate at all at this time and the needs of the individual should always be respected.

Other aspects

Although meditation is universal, there are other aspects of Buddhism it may well be useful to know about. Many Buddhists, for instance, would appreciate a visit from a Buddhist monk or sister. Buddhist monks and nuns are known as the members of a sangha (monastic order), and a monk is called a bhikku and a nun is a sister. The Buddhist Society or the London Buddhist Centre, plus many other organisations, will usually provide contacts quite swiftly. Many Buddhists share the prevailing British attitudes to their bodies, while others share those of the Indian sub-continent and will have strict rules of hygiene. Amongst these will be the requirement to wash before meditation and washing after defecation and urination (the patient may need help to do this). This is somewhat curious in view of the prevailing Buddhist view of the body as a temporary vessel, but it is by no means uncommon, and those who care for Buddhists should be sensitive to the possibility of there being such attitudes in the person or family concerned.

Many Buddhists are also vegetarian, although few go as far as the Jains in this matter. Some Buddhist groups, under Jain influence, will go out of their way to avoid killing even the smallest creature, such as an ant. Jainism is of the same generation as

Buddhism and its emphasis on not killing anything living has had an influence on some Buddhists of southern Indian schools.

Attitudes to life and death

Buddhism stresses the importance of relief of pain and suffering in general. However, a Buddhist who is dying usually does not wish to approach death with a clouded mind, and may be reluctant to take pain relieving drugs. This attitude is also often found amongst Buddhists who are ill but not necessarily dying. This is because of the Buddhist emphasis on mindfulness, meaning being aware of everything. It is often difficult for nurses and doctors to deal with this attitude to pain, even though it is by no means unique to Buddhism. Though it is still relatively uncommon in the West, this attitude to pain, fortitude and clarity has been increasing rapidly in its acceptability in recent years. A Buddhist or, indeed, any patient who refuses pain relief should not be bullied or cajoled by those who have been impressed, rightly, by what can be achieved by pain relief in a setting of modern palliative care. Instead, his views should be respected, with perhaps the only persuasion being to tell the patient that the drugs will not impair the senses, so that he knows that spiritual awareness is still possible after taking pain relieving drugs.

The attitude to life and death in Buddhism is different from that we are accustomed to in the West. It takes caring staff some time to get used to, but there is a famous Buddhist story which illustrates that Buddhists have been known to have some difficulty with it as well. It is called the story of Kisagotami and is taken from the parables of Buddhaghosha. (Buddhaghosha was a name used by several Buddhist writers.)

Kisagotami became in the family way and, when the 10 months were completed, gave birth to a son. When the boy was able to walk by himself, he died. The young girl, in her love for him, carried the dead child clasped to her bosom and went about from house to house asking if anyone would give her some medicine for it. When the neighbours saw this they said, 'Is the young girl mad that she carries about on her breast the dead body of her son!' But a wise man thinking to himself, 'Alas! This Kisagotami does not understand the law of death, I must comfort her,' said to her, 'My good girl, I cannot myself give medicine for it, but I know of a doctor who can attend to it.' The young girl said, 'If so, tell me who he is.' The wise man continued, 'Gautama can give medicine, you must go to him.'

Kisagotami went to Gautama and, doing homage to him, said, 'Lord and master, do you know any medicine that will be good for my boy?' Gautama replied, 'I know of some.' She asked, 'What medicine do you require?' He said, 'I want a handful of mustard seed.' The girl promised to procure it for him, but Gautama continued, 'I require some mustard seed taken from a house where no son, husband, parent, or slave has died.' The girl said, 'Very good,' and went to ask for some at the different houses, carrying the dead body of her son astride her hip. The people said, 'Here is some mustard seed, take it.' Then she asked, 'In my friend's house has there died a son, a husband, a parent, or a slave?' They replied, 'Lady, what is this that you say? The living are few, but the dead are many.' Then she went to other houses, but one said, 'I have lost a son'; another, 'I have lost my parents'; another, 'I have lost my slave.' At last, not being able to find a single house where no-one had died, from which to procure the mustard seed, she began to think, 'This is a heavy task that I am engaged in. I am not the only one whose son is dead. In the whole of the Savatthi country, everywhere children are dying, parents are dying.' Thinking thus, she acquired the law of fear and, putting away her affection for her child, she summoned up resolution and left the dead body in a forest; then she went to Gautama and paid him homage. He said to her, 'Have you procured the handful of mustard seed?' 'I have not,' she replied; 'the people of the village told me, "The living are few, but the dead are many."' Gautama said to her, 'You thought that you alone had lost a son; the law of death is that among all living creatures there is no permanence.' When Gautama had finished preaching the law, Kisagotami was established in the reward of Sotapatti; and all *the assembly who heard the law were also established in the reward of Sotapatti.*

Some time afterwards, when Kisagotami was one day engaged in the performance of her religious duties, she observed the lights in the houses now shining, now extinguished; and began to reflect, 'My state is like these lamps.' Gautama, who was then in the Gandhakuti building, sent his sacred appearance to her, which said to her, just as if he himself were preaching, 'All living beings resemble the flame of these lamps, one moment lighted, the next extinguished; those only who have arrived at Nirvana are at rest.' Kisagotami, on hearing this, reached the stage of a Rahanda possessed of intuitive knowledge.

The story illustrates the acceptance of the ordinary human life cycle and it is an attitude to be found amongst all schools of Buddhism, however much they vary in other respects. For this reason, Buddhists may accept impending death easily, often preferring to know so that they can prepare themselves, and may look towards their next life with apparent equanimity. The Buddhist acceptance of death may in fact be more striking than acceptance of pain. This can be difficult for caring staff to understand and work with.

After a Buddhist has died there is usually a cremation. It is conducted by a member of the family or by a Buddhist bhikku or sister. It is important that the body is wrapped in a sheet without emblems in order not to upset the surviving relatives, since consciousness is thought at this stage to be just departing the body.

Buddhists are usually very easy patients to care for at this time. The only word of caution is the need to be sensitive to all the different countries of origin, including the growing number of western Buddhists, as well as all the variant customs of the different Buddhist groups. However, it is comforting to remember that, while practices and ritual vary, attitudes to death do not. There is a calmness and acceptance of death amongst Buddhists from which others of us could undeniably learn. That calmness is something which caring staff are well placed to help to engender, by creating in the room or area of the ward a sense of calm and reflection in keeping with Buddhist meditative approaches.

9

Chinese beliefs and customs

As with all other groups, but especially in relation to people who are Chinese or of Chinese origin, it is essential not to generalise. China has a population of over one billion composed of five major ethnic groups. Some 6% of the population are non-Chinese. Expressed as a percentage that represents a small minority; numerically it accounts for some 60 million people. Religious groups are not as clearly differentiated as we in the West would expect them to be. Islam is the dominant religion in some regions; Christian communities have existed in China since the 16th century. Anti-religious feelings, based on the ideology of Marxist Maoism, are also prevalent. Since the Communists took power in 1949, and especially after the Cultural Revolution of 1966, attitudes to religion in China itself have been negative, often destructive, but have also led to a form of backlash in terms of increasing religious observance. Hong Kong, Macao and other Chinese populations have not been affected in the same way by the attack on the four 'Os' of old beliefs, old customs, old habits and old ideas. Whilst the Communist Government did not attack strongly the veneration of ancestors, a key part of Chinese faith, it was only the private, domestic aspects of ancestor veneration that did not suffer. The old ancestral halls, which were the clan temples and social and religious centres, were removed from clan control and turned into schools and social centres.

Religious beliefs

Broadly speaking, for the vast majority of people, if they practise any religion at all beyond the veneration of ancestors, the Chinese religious experience finds its 'philosophical' expression in a fusion of Confucianism, Taoism and Buddhism. A popular Chinese saying states 'Three religions – one religion', or 'Three paths to one and the same goal'. Suffice it to say, by way of illustrating this fusion, in most of South China it is hard to say where Taoism ends and Buddhism begins in relation to death and life-cycle events. It is also clearly common for Chinese Christians to practise some of the same rituals as their Buddhist and Taoist neighbours.

The separation of religion by class is also worth noting. In the past, the gentry and the scholars or mandarins, many of whom made up the core of the civil service, tended to be Confucian. Confucianism, in fact, is no religion as such. Unlike Taoism and Buddhism, it has neither priesthood nor temple. Its teachings are rooted in the Chinese reverence for the family system that has existed since time immemorial and for the moral education of the young within this system. Its concern is therefore with humanity's role in society, with both individual and social conduct. This includes being loyal and dutiful towards family, kin and neighbours, and respecting superiors and the aged. Beyond these aims, its concern is with norms of just government. The nation as an entirety is perceived as a family and, in pre-communist times, the emperor was regarded as father of the nation with similar paternal rights and duties towards his 'children' as are accorded to any elder of a family.

Taoism has its roots in the writings attributed to Lao-Tzu and stands in stark contrast to Confucianism. Society, power and wealth are seen as illusions. Humanity's task and duty are to develop inner self-hood and to live in harmony with the laws of Nature as manifested both in the inner and outer world. The enlightened adept is egoless, acting spontaneously without self-will or intended purpose. He is at one with the eternal, cosmic forces that govern Nature, including human nature itself. This mystical union with the cosmic totality makes him immortal. Chinese legend speaks of several sages who have attained such immortality and live in distant mountain fastnesses.

Confucianism and Taoism date from the 6th century BC. Buddhism arrived in China in the 1st century AD and has already been outlined in the previous chapter. In China, the popular appeal of Buddhism was immediate. One reason for this was the egalitarian Buddhist teaching that every human being was endowed with a Buddha-nature. The human soul by nature was likened to a perfect mirror; even though dust and dross may have dimmed its surface, given the effort, it could always be cleansed and made perfect again.

The 'three religions' have in common:

- a belief in the fundamental goodness of human nature
- a humanistic faith in self-improvement and spiritual enlightenment through training and learning
- the gods are seen as personifications of the forces of nature and as such impersonal powers. In the words of a Neo-Confucian sage of the 12th century: 'There is no man in Heaven who judges sins'
- none of the 'three religions' appeals to divine revelation in support for its teachings.

The Chinese perception of a cosmic harmony, wholeness and completeness does not allow for the absolute distinctions between opposites to which we are accustomed. Dualistic polarities – such as spirit and matter, good and evil, sacred and profane – tend to be perceived as complementing, rather than opposing, one another.

Chinese religious thought can be seen as a philosophical distillation essentially rooted in folk traditions millennia older than Confucianism and Taoism. Confucius himself claimed not to have said anything new in his teachings. He had merely summarised and made explicit ideas, precepts and customs that had previously been known and accepted.

Overall, what characterises Chinese religion is that, through the millennia of its evolution, it never entirely discarded earlier beliefs and practices when adopting new ones. That is why, in present day China, archaic rituals as well as highly evolved forms of belief can co-exist alongside one another, notwith-standing modern, atheistic ideologies such as Maoist Marxism. Chinese folk religion represents the earliest layer of Chinese ritual practices, supplemented and combined though they were with Taoism and Buddhism.

Veneration of ancestors

Key to all this is the attitude to ancestors. Respectful veneration of the dead is essential and death is not thought to sever the bonds of kinship. Unlike in the West, where psychologists and clergy now encourage people to work through their grief and accept separation, Chinese people behave in a different way – the relationship with the dead is just carried out differently. It is also very male. Although women provide the food offerings at the family shrine to the ancestors, the important sacrifices, essen-tial for the well-being of the ancestors both male and female, have to be made by sons.

Chinese people believe that a person has more than one soul and that, in accordance with the principles of yin and yang, one soul at least must be male and one female. When a person dies, the souls go different ways – the female sinks into the earth as a kwei (ghost) and disintegrates, whilst the male rises and becomes a shen (spirit). It is the shen that is the most important of the souls and requires all the special treatment, even though the kwei does not get neglected and still gets visited, especially during the Quing Ming festival when the graves are cleaned, incense is burned and the family have a kind of ceremonial picnic at the graveside. Shen souls reside – like all the others – in the spirit world after death, but they are also there in the tablets which families place on the family shrine.

Chinese people believe that the dead are judged and then punished. One soul, probably the shen, goes to Hell for a period (according to the length of the punishment) before moving to its allotted place in the spirit world. If that soul has access to plenty of money, it can use the money to bribe the official guards of Hell to get better treatment. However, wherever they end up, spirits need the same things as living men and women – food, clothes, shelter, money, status and veneration – hence the customs of offering food and the symbolic provision of all other necessities with paper replicas.

There are complications. Families are only responsible for their own dead. There is no communal responsibility for the spirits of those who had no sons. It used to be thought – and to some extent still is – that the spirits of those without children become hungry and malevolent ghosts. As a result, the Buddhists introduced a special ceremony – a public ceremony of propitiation where offerings are made to and for the childless dead. These ceremonies are not charitable in any sense – but merely offerings to stop the spirits becoming too nasty and malevolent. The ceremonies are held in the seventh lunar month, and still continue.

All this has led to a particular desire for sons amongst Chinese families – and the higher mortality rate for girls in China is well known. Other ways of dealing with the problem of childlessness have been found. Taoist monks and nuns elevate their deceased elders to the status of proper ancestors and provide them with food and veneration, whilst in some Chinese expatriate communities halls of faith – like the old clan halls – have been established to look after the childless elderly and to provide a more general ancestral respect for the dead, with the proper care of the death tablets of deceased members of the community.

In a sense this is a form of folk religion which crosses all religious boundaries and tends to unite Chinese people of all classes and origins. There is a kind of folklore alive with spirit gods, kitchen gods and earth gods. The gods have magical powers and are much feared, as well as being frequently bought off or placated. Festivals such as the Chinese New Year are closely tied in with folk religion – and practised by people who are Taoists, Confucians, Buddhists and even Christians despite the association with astrology, palm-reading, dream interpretation, soothsaying and magical practices.

Central to all Chinese folk religion is the family. It is in the family where the moral and ethical basis of society as a whole is thought to lie. Throughout Chinese history ancestors were worshipped and are respected even now. It is popularly believed that the spirits of ancestors are capable of punishing moral offenders as well as rewarding good behaviour. Belief in a continuity of life after death is a key part of all Chinese religions. Altars are built to ancestors and spirit tablets placed upon them. These can often be seen in the room of a dying person of a Chinese family.

Veneration of ancestors is universal amongst Chinese people across all religious divides. Some bigoted Chinese Christians may cheerfully refer to Taoism and Buddhism as 'devil worship' – a strange description of the followers of Buddha and Confucius – but, despite religious enmity, they may still follow the same rituals of ancestor worship as their non-Christian neighbours.

Preparing for death

An impending death is accepted as a natural event for which one wishes to be prepared. As soon as it becomes clear that a person is unlikely to recover, he will be told and a coffin procured. Often coffins are purchased much earlier in life by children wanting to show their parents that everything will be done properly when the time comes. It is not uncommon for the dying person to be in the room with his own coffin. Prayers and blessings will be said. Indeed, everything will be done to convey to the dying person that everyone is mindful that for him the most important thing in life, now ending fast, is to be buried properly with all the necessary dignity, pomp and circumstance. There are few universal rituals to be performed during the process of dying. However, the concern for propriety after death is universal and paramount.

Customs and ceremonies surrounding death

A dying Chinese person may want to see the Buddhist priest or sister – often to discuss funeral arrangements and to make sure that the family will be gathered around. A Christian may want to see a priest for much the same purpose.

Once death has taken place, the body is washed by the family in special water, thought to be protected by a guardian spirit, an uneven number of times. The ceremony is known as 'buying the water'. As in other religions, the feeling that the body can become in some way possessed by demonic spirits is very strong: as a precaution incense is burned and firecrackers set off.

Before it is dressed, the body is covered in wadding – another way of keeping the spirits out. The clothing is usually cotton – unless the family is very wealthy in which case silk may be used. The garments have no buttons or zips, but are tied with fabric ties so that the clothing looks rather like those worn by a Buddhist priest.

Before he dies, the dying person may ask to see the garments, including socks and shoes, in order to check that they are in keeping with his status and the solemnity of his death. Men have a head-dress similar to that of a Buddhist priest, whilst women, their hair piled high and dressed with gold or jade, wear the seven-cornered 'Lotus flower hat'. The men often have a jade snuff bottle put in the tomb with them. The practice of having jade near the body dates from a very early period.

After being dressed, the body is bound at the feet with a piece of rope to stop it leaping about if it is attacked by evil spirits. It is then laid out on the bed for family and friends to pay their last respects. A drummer is positioned outside the door – on the left-hand side for a man, on the right for a woman – and is required to play warning beats as guests approach in order to ensure that the family can be found in suitable, formal tableau style attitudes of mourning.

The coffin is placed on two stools, head pointing to the door, and a table bearing five vases and two candlesticks is arranged to serve as an altar. There are blue and white paper flowers in the vases; the two candlesticks are lit at night. Alongside these objects is a pagoda-shaped stand bearing a bowl of sesame oil on which floats a burning wick of twisted cotton. In the centre of the altar next to the coffin is the spirit tablet into which one of the deceased person's souls has entered and on which his name is inscribed. Ordinarily, the food for the bereaved family is standard; but when guests come a banquet is provided. Guests often bring some of the food themselves to ensure an abundant spread. Once again, the dying person often wishes to be assured that such a banquet will take place, even in a community where there are few Chinese people.

It is customary for the guests to bring gifts for the deceased. Such gifts include money in a yellow paper envelope with a strip of blue to indicate mourning. There are also banners which bear the words 'May the soul return to the Western Heaven'. These will be carried in the funeral procession and burned after the service of committal. Then there is gold and silver paper money and paper carts and horses – all for burning in the final cortege.

Before the burial, specialists have to be consulted. The religious authorities will assess the family's wealth and decide just how many masses need to be sung in order to gain entrance to the Western Heaven. The virtues of the dead person are chanted aloud. If the deceased was notoriously an evil-doer, the priests have to make intercessions on his behalf, a form of plea in mitigation, imploring the bad spirits to release the soul of their client. One of the 'adepts' (experts) will determine the best site for the burial and the diviner is called in to get the spirits of those already buried in the graveyard to agree on the siting.

After the masses for the dead person have been sung, the family prepares paper offerings representing the things the person was involved with during his lifetime. In this way servants, cars, carts, horses, rickshaws and suchlike made of paper are prepared for the deceased's use in the nether world society. On the eve of the funeral these paper objects are taken out and burned. Once again, an attendant is there beating at the bonfire with a long pole to keep any lurking evil spirits away. Often boiled rice and water are also scattered to distract the attention of the Hungry Ghosts.

On the morning of the funeral, the body is taken out head first. The youngest son breaks a drinking vessel at its head for use by the deceased in the nether world. Then there is a proper funeral procession, grouped in multiples of eight; there are banners with eulogies about the deceased, lanterns, flowers and other objects. At intervals along the route, paper money is thrown in the air to distract malignant spirits.

Once the procession arrives at the cemetery, the coffin is lowered into the grave. The diviner assures the relatives that the place is suitable. The mourners weep and wail by the graveside, each scattering a handful of earth onto the coffin. As the weeping dies down, a bonfire is made of the paper articles and the ceremony comes to an end. Mourning, however, continues and every dying Chinese person would want this to be so.

The ceremonies afterwards last for at least the next 24 hours and are repeated on various auspicious days in the ensuing year. Guests are always welcome at any of these ceremonies. Friends of different background and culture are keenly encouraged to join the mourning. It is thought that the presence of someone who is not Chinese and not a member of the family gives 'face' (importance) to the deceased and brings honour to the bereaved family.

It is, of course, always advisable to check first that an outsider would be welcome, but Chinese patients receiving palliative and terminal care often mention that they would welcome the presence of staff who had cared for them both at the funeral and the feast at the house.

As can be seen, for many Chinese people death and dying are taken as the culmination of the religious life. A proper death and funeral are of paramount importance – hence the concern with the funeral arrangements and the nature of the coffin. For caring staff it is important to realise that this is not a morbid obsession, but a key part of religious faith: a person who has not had a proper funeral has not lived properly. By the same token, if a person cannot trust his family to provide him with all the ceremonies of honour at his death, how can he take their grief during his final illness seriously? These are concerns often voiced at the bedside of a terminally ill Chinese man (more often by a man than by a woman). He wants to know that everything has been organised and to check that the family knows and remembers what to do.

There will be a great deal of variation in the ritual that is to be undertaken, but in almost all cases the washing, the insistence on burial, the requirement of feasting and formal mourning will be the same. (In Hong Kong exhumation takes place after six years and the bones are kept in a funerary jar.)

For caring staff, the most helpful thing, as ever, is to encourage the dying person to talk about his concerns and worries: about what will happen to his body and soul, the difficulties to be encountered on the journey to the Western Heaven. At the same time, it is important for the carer to realise that these concerns may be mixed in with other religious beliefs, notably those of Buddhism and Christianity which are described elsewhere in this book. It is the mixture of religious and social customs that is so bewildering for caring staff when looking after Chinese patients. Anyone brought up in the attitudes of western Christianity, which regards itself as one single faith, may find this difficult to take on board unless prepared to expect it.

10

Japanese beliefs and customs

Religions

The traditional religion of Japan is Shintoism, but Buddhism, Confucianism and Taoism also have a presence in Japan and amongst Japanese people. To add to all these, Christianity has a relatively minor presence, as well as the new religions, or cults, which are strong in parts of Japan and spreading to parts of the West. Some of the new religions (Shinko Shukyo) date to the early 19th century. Others are newer, established by people who feel a form of divine revelation, set up a religious grouping and allow relatively easy entry for the followers they attract.

Although Shintoism is the oldest religion, and the grandest, in Japan, Buddhism is probably the most common. It is often the case that a Japanese house will have a shrine for the Shinto gods (a kamidana) alongside a Buddha altar (a butsudan). When Japanese people marry they often have the union blessed by a Shinto ceremony. On the other hand, for a funeral, it is often the Buddhist monks who are called. However, what crosses all sectarian lines is the deep-seated veneration of ancestors, similar to that found amongst Chinese people.

The Shinto religion

Shinto is the word used in the West for the Japanese term Kami-no-Michi, the way of the gods (kami). It is a mixture of ancient beliefs, but its main centre appears to be an emphasis on perfection, cleanliness and harmony with nature. The emphasis on ritual purity is intense. Some scholars have suggested that the desire to leave funeral rites to Buddhist monks rather than carry them out themselves may be because Shinto priests are so concerned at the pollution that will adhere to them through contact with the dead. (There is a sense of pollution from the dead that runs through many religions – it is similar to the prohibition in Judaism applied to the priests [those called Cohen or from a priestly family] from entering a cemetery and being at a funeral.)

There are three elements to the universe – humanity, nature and the kami. Although the kami are usually translated into English as spirits or gods, they are actually rather different. They are linked with ancestors and inhabit the heavens, the underworld and various other places. Some are attached to particular clans, others to particular activities. Their help is sought at shrines through prayer and offerings.

Death is an evil that must be accepted. After death, the spirits move into a place no longer pure, with decay and corruption rife. However, then, through family effort, they are finally released from physical limitations and become part of the life force and do not necessarily remain totally out of contact with family. The dead remain close to the living, as in Chinese belief.

Shinto rituals provide the dead with a way of escaping complete disintegration. Through festivals for the deceased (matsuri), the dead escape impurity, become exalted as spirits and eventually become part of the world of the kami. Having been rescued from disintegration, these spirits can watch over their families and help them with blessings and guidance. The family continues to venerate their ancestors, thanking them for their protection and bringing them gifts and prayer, rather as in Chinese custom and as carried out by Japanese from other faiths as well.

The souls of the dead (tamishii) can be restless and appear in many forms, including monsters and bright lights. These need to be placated. This restlessness is particularly strong amongst those who have died violent deaths – it is for this reason that small shrines are so often to be found at the roadside where accidents have taken place in Japan.

The appeasement of the soul is considered an essential role of the family. The act of appeasement is called chinkon, an act of private meditation, and it must be carried out at least for the 49 days the soul of the deceased is supposed to linger in the house. If all is done properly, the tamishii becomes a kami after 33 years and reaches complete happiness.

Shinto funerals

These are very uncommon because of concerns about ritual purity, as explained above. However, a Shinto funeral is always held for Shinto priests, for important Shinto believers and for the Imperial family. The ritual is simple and beautiful. It starts at home, where the dead person has been washed, dressed and placed in the coffin. The chief mourner urges the evil spirits to depart and purifies the house, and everyone present, with a sprinkling of salt water. Then the spirit of the departed is asked to enter the small shrine (tamashiro) which holds the tablet on which his or her name has been inscribed. Purification, prayer and a sacred meal follow, and the funeral ends with prayers that ask for the soul to survive and for it to rest in peace, before burial or cremation.

Some Japanese homes have small private shrines in their gardens, which, if they are Shinto shrines, contain symbols of the local kami and what is called a taima at the centre, a board from the main Shinto shrine at Ise which represents the universal kami. A small box containing the memorial tablets of deceased members of the family, plus a mirror, stand on top.

Japanese customs: the Bon festival

Each summer, people leave the cities for their home towns for the Bon festival, which is a time for celebrating and consoling the spirits of the dead. This festival, which really only occurs still in small towns and villages, was introduced to Japan by the Buddhists. It is somewhat like the secular, commercialised version of Hallowe'en, except that it is serious and really emphasises the closeness of the dead to the living, something western religions have found difficult and have often classed as superstition.

When spirits return to their former homes for the Bon festival, there is huge celebration and welcome. There is a welcoming fire (mukaebi), offerings are placed on the household altar and there is feasting galore. Two days later, there is a sending off fire (okuribi) which guides the spirits back to their spiritual homes. In some places fires are replaced by lighting candles and floating them down the rivers, which is beautiful. People use the Bon festival to consult the sprits about important business and family matters, without which things would go less well.

11

Humanism

In previous editions of this book, a separate section on humanism seemed unnecessary. Since the book is about caring for people of different faiths, and humanists argue energetically that theirs is not a faith, leaving out humanism seemed logical. However, there have been some changes since the early 1980s when this book first appeared.

Firstly, the rise in the number and different types of green (conservationist) and humanist funerals has grown exponentially, suggesting a new phenomenon amongst those who were formerly spirituality denying agnostics or atheists. People who have no particular religious faith nevertheless want to express something spiritual at the time of a death of a loved one. The traditions of the 'old' faiths will not do. For some of these people, humanism as previously understood will not do either – too spare, too dry, too rational. However, for others it is exactly what they want – a human centred, grief acknowledging, next world denying way of coping with death.

Consequently, this chapter deals both with the traditional humanist view and the more modern approaches.

Traditional humanist view

The traditional form of humanism has its origins with the Greek philosophers such as Protagoras (c 480–410 BC), Democritus (c 460–360 BC) and Epicurus (341–271 BC). These thinkers taught that 'man is the measure of all things'. On death, Epicurus taught that it is simply the end of life, and the epitaphs of his followers were often inscribed with the words:

I was not – I have been – I am not – I do not mind.

For humanists, death is just a simple fact – the marvellous machine that is the human body simply wears out, or is affected by disease which human beings have not yet learned to cure. There is no plague sent by gods, illness is not a punishment, tragedies are just the way of the world and we must all die.

In some ways, this is a comforting and comfortable doctrine. There is no fear of what might happen in the afterlife. In Greek thought, Hades was inevitable, a grey and shady place, rather than a hell, a place of punishment. Humanists are either true atheists or agnostics. Either way, their world is very much centred on humanity, with a moral imperative – for humanism has a strong moral code – on doing what one can for fellow human beings.

However, there is a catch. Many modern humanists are also utilitarians, believing that society should aim for the greatest happiness of the greatest number of people. Actions are right or wrong depending on whether they decrease or increase human happiness. Thus, with the contemporary debate over euthanasia or assisted suicide, most humanists place themselves in the camp in favour of help with suicide for terminally ill people, on the grounds that it brings greater happiness to the people concerned and to those around them, if all agree. The sense that doctors, by aiding such a suicide, might in some way be committing a sin is one that is incomprehensible to many humanists, based as it is on a belief in human life as divine creation there for God, rather than human beings, to give or take away.

Other approaches

Not all humanists fit this rather traditional, logical, this-world centred view. There are many people who have a sense of the spiritual which has no religious home. In any philosophical sense, they are humanists because they have no belief in a divine or 'other' being. The supernatural is not something they believe in. Yet, alongside their lack of belief in a deity goes a strong sense of wishing to have spiritual ceremonies, lighting candles, holding hands, gaining strength from the support of other human beings. Some of this has its roots in the person centred psychotherapies – human strength comes from self-understanding and human support. However, some has its roots in a yearning for ritual without the certainty – or even probability – of belief. Hence we are seeing rituals growing up that have no deity, no belief pattern, behind them. The marking of the new moon, for instance, can be linked with women's spirituality or with traditional witchcraft, wicca. Equally, it can be a ritual that gives meaning to those who have no such rituals in their lives. Wesley Carr has described the character of contemporary atheism as being *very different from earlier forms*. It is fashionable to be interested in the spiritual. There is the rise in New Age philosophies which appear to be agnostic whilst emphasising the personal and the spiritual. A longing for some kind of spiritual reference point and understanding without turning to established religious forms seems widespread.

Funerals

Similarly, with funerals, there is a huge variety of humanistic approaches, from the strongly green, conservationist, funerals in woodland with cardboard coffins for ecological reasons, to the more staid cremations with a solemn address reciting the good deeds of the person who has died, without asking for peace for his or her soul.

Green funerals are growing in popularity and a consciousness of death is often a part of that approach. Increasingly, people are buying their cardboard coffins in advance and decorating them themselves.

Whichever kind of humanist funeral is to take place, most will have five sections, similar to many religious funerals. There will be:

- words of welcome
- a few songs and readings about death and life and perhaps some readings which were favourites of the person who has died
- an address reciting the virtues of the person
- the consignment of the coffin to the earth or the furnace
- a closing ceremony in which the person officiating will thank people for coming and ask that the memory of the person who has died might strengthen the lives of those still alive – the nearest humanists get to a sense of immortality.

Approaches to death and bereavement

Though there are variants, and though there is a growing interest in mysticism amongst humanists, without a deity at its core, most humanists have simple approaches to death and to bereavement and will not wish for any secrets to be withheld, or for any pain relief available to be withheld at any time. For most humanists, suffering itself is anathema and in no sense ennobling.

Humanists are usually easy to care for in the spiritual sense – precisely because of their lack of formal belief and their reliance on human support. There are, obviously, no humanist chaplains, although Unitarian ministers will often visit humanists on request. Equally, the Humanist societies to which many belong will often provide people for dying patients to talk to – counsellors, philosophical guides and so on. For those more involved in New Age philosophies, there are usually friends and leaders who will come and give support as needed, though often the Unitarian chaplain will help if required.

The only issue that can arise with humanists being cared for at the end of their lives is a sense of urgency about doing a variety of things, in part because of the very certainty that this is the end. Though other patients frequently want to finish something off, or see some grandchild born, or whatever, humanists are often more urgent about such things and more determined to get things done. If everything is in this life, if how we are remembered is to be judged purely by what is achieved in the real world, in this world, then trying to achieve yet more in the last weeks or months of life is understandable – though it can make caring for people with that sense of urgency difficult.

Most humanists will not be like this, however. They will be quiet and resigned and will enjoy conversations on the subject of their belief and what will happen after their deaths. The main problems arise when the person dying is a humanist and the family, or chief carers, are something else and want a different kind of funeral. However, that is as true of people of other faiths too – families do not always follow the wishes of their dear departed, particularly if they do not share the faith and life approach that he held.

12

People as individuals

All the preceding sections of this book have been a broad guide as to what to do in given situations, with some basic information about different belief systems. This guide will by no means cover all eventualities, nor will it answer every question. It may, however, suggest at least to some extent what the questions might be and give some guidance as to when they are likely to occur.

What is without doubt, however, is that the caring nurse's interest and attempt to know something about the patient's religious and cultural background give enormous support, not only to the patient, but also to family and friends.

Families find it helpful and supportive to find caring staff who do not regard them as 'peculiar' or 'strange' and who have taken the trouble to learn something of their customs and beliefs. It makes an enormous difference to the relationships between nurses, family, friends and the patient if this can be the case, and would be valuable for that alone – if that were all that was achieved.

In fact, understanding something about the patient's religious and cultural background contributes far more to the caring process. Instead of apparently tending purely to the physical needs of the patient – and no nurse really does just that – the psychological needs, the emotional needs and the spiritual needs are all being taken into account. The physical needs are in any case partly shaped by those other needs, but the terminally ill patient requires care of the whole person even more than the acutely ill, but non-terminal, patient.

Spiritual needs

First of all, spiritual needs are often very obvious. Patients and families make them very clear, but the problem hitherto has been in the caring staff's lack of skill and training in recognising those needs. The signs of emotional distress, desire to fulfil religious ritual, concern with the customs of particular cultural or religious groups and a desire to somehow make one's peace with the world, and make amends with those one thinks one has harmed or offended, are all possible indicators of spiritual need and longings. Sometimes concern with making peace with God and human beings is stronger than worry about pain or discomfort. Sometimes a desire to perform a ritual is more important than the need to be washed or to take drugs.

Caring for the individual

The reason for this is obvious in one way. Making one's peace with one's maker or whatever psychospiritual powers one believes exist – if one believes at all – becomes paramount amongst those who are terminally ill. This is not to over-dramatise the situation, but to point out that, in caring for the terminally ill, spiritual urgency has to be taken into account. Within that urgency are to be found conflicts about deeds done and not sorted out with other human beings and the divine, and deeds not done, which one would have liked to have done, including those which might be regarded as wrong or sinful in one's own religious or moral framework. In their relationships with terminally ill patients, nurses and other caring staff may find themselves having to deal with these conflicts – and, in many cases, these conflicts have a major negative component with which most nurses have no experience in dealing. Conventional religious patterns of confession, prayer, absolution and

asking forgiveness of human beings are all part of this phenomenon, but they are by no means the whole.

With this in mind nurses, who are sitting with patients, trying
to bring them comfort and asking them about their needs and
desires, need to think that part of what may emerge may be
highly negative and very difficult, but that the very expression
of it may well bring relief to some of the patients. It may also be
possible to help others by asking clergy of their own faith to
visit, or psychologists with skills in this kind of area. The very
private relationship that nurses have with their patients, when
they have looked after them for a long time, often enables them
to pick up some of these conflicts, difficulties and desires even
when speech has become problematic. Comfort, in the form of
hugs, physical touch and speech, can bring relief. However,
more may be wanted and the sensitive nurse, who knows a little
about the emotions that can be present in patients near the end
of life, can be enormously helpful in bringing about some kind
of emotional and psychospiritual resolution – even if it is only
partial. That sensitivity may include the offering of a crucifix to a
Catholic patient, or giving a Muslim patient water for washing.
It might mean providing Ganges water for a Hindu, or reading a
psalm to a Jew. An awareness of religious holidays helps as well.
A nurse who goes up to a Muslim patient and says 'I know it is
your Id today – would you like an Imam to come in?' has
acknowledged the individuality of that patient and made him or
her aware that those festivals are important on the nurse's
calendar – because of the patient. In a hospice setting, this would
no longer be unusual. In a busy hospital, this might be a marker
that the needs of religious and cultural minorities are being
taken seriously and seen as being as important, proportionately,
as the festivals of the dominant groups.

The more general message is important too. In the first edition
of this book, I wrote that:

> Many members of religious minorities find that hospitals are
> still too 'Christian', too unaware of their needs.

That has not changed greatly in Britain, though there are some
hospitals and hospices which have made a major effort. One

interfaith hospice now operates for inpatients in London, and several US hospitals have made sterling advances in reaching out to some particular groups, notably Hispanic Catholics with different customs, and black Muslims. Nevertheless, there is still much to be done to decrease the sense of disaffection from public institutions such as hospitals amongst ethnic and religious minority groups. The demonstration of knowledge, albeit limited, understanding, interest and, above all, an awareness of and sensitivity to special needs can do much to counter that sense of disaffection. Although that sense of dissatisfaction is not always justified, nevertheless it is true to say that when a member of a religious or ethnic minority states that staff in a particular caring institution have done little to understand their customs, that is probably at least partially true.

No book can provide all the information caring staff might find useful. This book does not even attempt to do so. What it does, however, is to try to give some basic guidelines. Those having been taken into account, the best advice is to ask the patient and the family and show that staff care about their needs. No-one ever minds being asked about their customs and beliefs, if the subject is approached with genuine interest and politeness. Indeed, the reverse is true – such interest is welcomed and enjoyed. In the case of terminally ill patients, those rituals, beliefs and customs often take on great importance. Awareness of, and sensitivity to, those requirements will be much appreciated. Sensitivity to these issues will bring genuine comfort, support and help to those whose need for it is often very great indeed.

General information and bibliography

Useful addresses

Hospital Chaplaincies Council
Church House
Great Smith Street
London SW1P 3NZ
Tel: 020 7898 1894
Fax: 020 7898 1891

National Council for Hospice and Specialist Palliative
Care Services
34–44 Britannia Street
London WC1X 9JG
Tel: 020 7520 8299

Hospice Information Service
St Christopher's Hospice
51–59 Lawrie Park Road
London SE26 6DZ
Tel: 020 8778 9252

Cruse Bereavement Care
Cruse House
126 Sheen Road
Richmond
Surrey TW9 1UR
Tel: 020 8940 4818
Helpline: 020 8332 7227

The Buddhist Hospice Trust
Website: www.buddhisthospice.org.uk

CancerBACUP
3 Bath Place
Rivington Street
London EC2A 3DR
Tel: 020 7696 9003
Helpline: 0808 800 1234

Bibliography

General interest

Ainsworth-Smith I and Speck P (1982) *Letting Go: caring for the dying and bereaved*. SPCK, London.

Arora S, Coker N, Gillam S *et al.* (2000) *Improving the Health of Black and Minority Ethnic Groups: a guide for primary care organisations*. King's Fund, London.

Carr AW (1974) Contemporary non-theistic spirituality. *Theology*. **77**(650): 412–17.

Clark J (2003) Patient centred death. *BMJ*. **327**: 174–5.

Cobb M and Robshaw V (eds) (1998) *The Spiritual Challenge of Health Care*. Churchill Livingstone, Edinburgh.

Davie G (1994) *Religion in Britain since 1945. Believing without belonging*. Blackwell, Oxford.

Dinnage R (1990) *The Ruffian on The Stair*. Viking, London.

Enright DJ (1983) *The Oxford Book of Death*. Oxford University Press, Oxford.

Gittings C (1984) *Death, Burial and the Individual in Early Modern Britain*. Croon Helm, London.

Green J (1991) Death with dignity: meeting the spiritual needs of patients in a multi-cultural society. *Nursing Times*. Macmillan Magazines, London.

Hinton J (1972) *Dying* (2e). Penguin, Harmondsworth.

Howarth G and Leaman O (eds) (2001) *Encyclopedia of Death and Dying*. Routledge, London.

Jupp P and Gittings C (1999) *Death in England: an illustrated history*. Manchester University Press, Manchester.

Lee E (2002) *In Your Own Time: a guide for patients and their carers facing a last illness at home*. Oxford University Press, Oxford.

Lewis CS (1961) *A Grief Observed*. Faber, London.

Noll P (1989) *In the Face of Death*. Viking, London and New York.

Nuland S (1994) *How We Die*. Alfred A Knopf, New York.

Parkes CM (1975) *Bereavement: studies of grief in adult life*. Penguin, Harmondsworth.

Silverman PR (2000) *Never Too Young to Know: death in children's lives*. Oxford University Press, Oxford.

Smart N (1989) *The World's Religions*. Cambridge University Press, Cambridge.

Taylor T (2002) *The Buried Soul: how humans invented death*. Fourth Estate, London.

Thomas K (2003) *Caring for the Dying at Home*. Radcliffe Medical Press, Oxford.

Walter T (1994) *The Revival of Death*. Routledge, London.

Walter T (2003) Historical and cultural variants on the good death. *BMJ*. **327**: 218–20.

Waterhouse M (2003) *Staying Close: a positive approach to dying and bereavement*. Constable, London.

Young M and Cullen L (1996) *A Good Death – conversations with East Londoners*. Routledge, London.

Specific interest

Burkhardt VR (1982) *Chinese Creeds and Customs*. South China Morning Post, Hong Kong.

Firth S (2001) *Wider Horizons: care of the dying in a multicultural society*. National Council for Hospice and Specialist Palliative Care Services, London.

Gatrad AR, Brown E, Notta H et al. (2003) Palliative care needs of minorities. BMJ. **327**: 176–7.

Harvey P (1990) An Introduction to Buddhism. Cambridge University Press, Cambridge.

Henley A (1982–84) Asians in Britain (3 vols). Caring for Sikhs and their Families: religious aspects of care. Caring for Muslims and their Families: religious aspects of care. Caring for Hindus and their Families: religious aspects of care. DHSS and King Edward's Hospital Fund for London, National Extension College, London.

Iqbal M (1981) East Meets West (3e). Commission for Racial Equality, London.

Locke DC (1982) Increasing Multicultural Understanding – a comprehensive model. Sage Publications, California.

Lothian Community Relations Council (1984) Religions and Cultures: a guide to patients' beliefs and customs for health service staff. Lothian Community Relations Council, Edinburgh.

McGilloway O and Myco F (eds) (1985) Nursing and Spiritual Care. Harper and Row, London.

Neuberger J and White J (eds) (1991) A Necessary End. Macmillan, London.

Orchard H (ed.) (2001) Spirituality in Health Care Contexts. Jessica Kingsley Publishers, London.

Raft: The Journal of the Buddhist Hospice Trust. Spring 2003 (no. 23). Newport, Isle of Wight.

Rees D (1997) Death and Bereavement – the psychological, religious and cultural interfaces. Whurr Publishers, London.

Riemer J (ed.) (1995) Jewish Insights on Death and Mourning. Schocken Books, New York.

Sampson C (1982) The Neglected Ethic: religious and cultural factors in the care of patients. McGraw-Hill, Maidenhead.

Saunders C, Summers DH and Teller N (1981) Hospice, The Living Idea. Edward Arnold, London.

Sheikh A and Gatrad AR (2000) Caring for Muslim Patients. Radcliffe Medical Press, Oxford.

Sue DW and Sue D (1990) Counselling the Culturally Different; theory and practice (2e). John Wiley, New York.

Wieseltier L (1998) Kaddish. Macmillan, London.

Index